D.H. William M.D.
Sept 1996

Group Therapy for
Schizophrenic Patients

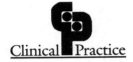

Clinical Practice

Number 39

Judith H. Gold, M.D., F.R.C.P.C.
Elissa P. Benedek, M.D.
Series Editors

Group Therapy for Schizophrenic Patients

Nick Kanas, M.D.
Professor and Director
Group Therapy Training Program
Department of Psychiatry
University of California, San Francisco

Assistant Chief
Psychiatry Service
Department of Veterans Affairs Medical Center
San Francisco, California

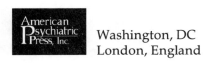

Washington, DC
London, England

Copyright © 1996 American Psychiatric Press, Inc.
ALL RIGHTS RESERVED
Manufactured in the United States of America on acid-free paper
First Edition   99   98   97   96   4   3   2   1

American Psychiatric Press, Inc.
1400 K Street, N.W., Washington, DC 20005

Library of Congress Cataloging-in-Publication Data
Group therapy for schizophrenic patients / [edited by] Nick Kanas.
     p.   cm. — (Clinical practice series ; #39)
    Includes bibliographical references and index.
    ISBN 0-88048-172-2 (alk. paper)
    1. Schizophrenia—Treatment.   2. Group psychotherapy.   I. Kanas,
Nick, 1945–   .   II. Series: Clinical practice ; no. 39.
    [DNLM: 1. Schizophrenia—therapy.   2. Psychotherapy, Group.   W1
CL767J no.39 1996 / WM 203 G882 1996]
RC514.G75   1996
616.89'820651—dc20
DNLM/DLC
for Library of Congress   96-4745
                                                    CIP

British Library Cataloguing in Publication Data
A CIP record is available from the British Library.

Contents

List of Tables

About the Author

*D*r. Kanas has been leading therapy groups involving schizo-phrenic patients for more than 20 years. He has written more than 70 papers, books, and book chapters on group therapy and small group behavior. Populations he has studied include schizo-phrenic, alcoholic, bipolar, and posttraumatic stress disorder patients; mental health staff and trainees; and astronauts and cosmonauts. Currently, Dr. Kanas is a Fellow of both the American Psychiatric Association and the American Group Psychotherapy Association, and he is a psychiatric evaluator for the NASA astronaut selection program. In addition to his ongoing group therapy work, he is the principal investigator of both a small group space simulation study conducted in Moscow and a study involving the interactions of astronauts and cosmonauts in space.

Introduction
to the Clinical Practice Series

Over the years of its existence the series of monographs entitled *Clinical Insights* gradually became focused on providing current, factual, and theoretical material of interest to the clinician working outside of a hospital setting. To reflect this orientation, the name of the Series has been changed to *Clinical Practice.*

The Clinical Practice Series will provide books that give the mental health clinician a practical, clinical approach to a variety of psychiatric problems. These books will provide up-to-date literature reviews and emphasize the most recent treatment methods. Thus, the publications in the Series will interest clinicians working both in psychiatry and in the other mental health professions.

Each year a number of books will be published dealing with all aspects of clinical practice. In addition, from time to time when appropriate, the publications may be revised and updated. Thus, the Series will provide quick access to relevant and important areas of psychiatric practice. Some books in the Series will be authored by a person considered to be an expert in that particular area; others will be edited by such an expert, who will also draw together other knowledgeable authors to produce a comprehensive overview of that topic.

Some of the books in the Clinical Practice Series will have their foundation in presentations at an annual meeting of the American Psychiatric Association. All will contain the most recently available information on the subjects discussed. Theoretical and scientific data will be applied to clinical situations, and case illustrations will be utilized in order to make the material even more relevant for the practitioner. Thus, the Clinical Practice Series should provide educational reading in a compact format especially designed for the mental health clinician–psychiatrist.

Judith H. Gold, M.D., F.R.C.P.C.
Series Editor

Clinical Practice Series Titles

Group Therapy for Schizophrenic Patients (#39)
By Nick Kanas, M.D.

Sexual Harassment in the Workplace and Academia: Psychiatric
Issues (#38)
Edited by Diane K. Shrier, M.D.

Use of Neuroleptics in Children (#37)
Edited by Mary Ann Richardson, Ph.D., and Gary Haugland, M.A.

The New Pharmacotherapy of Schizophrenia (#36)
Edited by Alan Breier, M.D.

Clinical Assessment and Management of Severe Personality
Disorders (#35)
Edited by Paul S. Links, M.D., M.Sc., F.R.C.P.C.

Predictors of Treatment Response in Mood Disorders (#34)
Edited by Paul J. Goodnick, M.D.

Successful Psychiatric Practice in Changing Times: Current
Dilemmas, Choices, and Solutions (#33)
Edited by Edward K. Silberman, M.D.

Alternatives to Hospitalization for Acute Psychiatric Treatment (#32)
Edited by Richard Warner, M.B., D.P.M.

Behavioral Complications in Alzheimer's Disease (#31)
Edited by Brian A. Lawlor, M.D.

Patient Violence and the Clinician (#30)
Edited by Burr S. Eichelman, M.D., Ph.D., and
Anne C. Hartwig, J.D., Ph.D.

Effective Use of Group Therapy in Managed Care (#29)
Edited by K. Roy MacKenzie, M.D., F.R.C.P.C.

Rediscovering Childhood Trauma: Historical Casebook and Clinical
Applications (#28)
Edited by Jean M. Goodwin, M.D., M.P.H.

Treatment of Adult Survivors of Incest (#27)
Edited by Patricia L. Paddison, M.D.

Madness and Loss of Motherhood: Sexuality, Reproduction, and Long-Term Mental Illness (#26)
Edited by Roberta J. Apfel, M.D., M.P.H., and
Maryellen H. Handel, Ph.D.

Psychiatric Aspects of Symptom Management in Cancer Patients (#25)
Edited by William Breitbart, M.D., and Jimmie C. Holland, M.D.

Responding to Disaster: A Guide for Mental Health Professionals (#24)
Edited by Linda S. Austin, M.D.

Psychopharmacological Treatment Complications in the Elderly (#23)
Edited by Charles A. Shamoian, M.D., Ph.D.

Anxiety Disorders in Children and Adolescents (#22)
By Syed Arshad Husain, M.D., F.R.C.P.C., F.R.C.Psych., and
Javad Kashani, M.D.

Suicide and Clinical Practice (#21)
Edited by Douglas Jacobs, M.D.

Special Problems in Managing Eating Disorders (#20)
Edited by Joel Yager, M.D., Harry E. Gwirtsman, M.D., and
Carole K. Edelstein, M.D.

Children and AIDS (#19)
Edited by Margaret L. Stuber, M.D.

Current Treatments of Obsessive-Compulsive Disorder (#18)
Edited by Michele Tortora Pato, M.D., and Joseph Zohar, M.D.

Benzodiazepines in Clinical Practice: Risks and Benefits (#17)
Edited by Peter P. Roy-Byrne, M.D., and Deborah S. Cowley, M.D.

Adolescent Psychotherapy (#16)
Edited by Marcia Slomowitz, M.D.

Family Approaches in Treatment of Eating Disorders (#15)
Edited by D. Blake Woodside, M.D., M.Sc., F.R.C.P.C., and
Lorie Shekter-Wolfson, M.S.W., C.S.W.

Clinical Management of Gender Identity Disorders in Children and Adults (#14)
Edited by Ray Blanchard, Ph.D., and Betty W. Steiner, M.B., F.R.C.P.C.

Preface

Schizophrenia is a serious mental illness that produces disruptions in thought, mood, and behavior. It afflicts 1% of the population worldwide. In the United States alone, some three million people will experience the pain and suffering of this severe, chronic illness, and millions more of their family and friends will be indirectly affected. Although antipsychotic medications generally are considered to be the primary treatment intervention for this condition, these drugs are not cures. Many patients fail to respond adequately, and even those who do respond have side effects and continue to experience psychosocial problems. There is a critical need for new treatment approaches that are safe and that will help these patients deal effectively with their inner and outer worlds.

In controlled studies, group therapy has been found to be a useful adjunct to medications in helping schizophrenic patients cope with their illness and relate better with others. However, like any potent treatment, therapy groups can be harmful if used incorrectly by individuals who are not aware of potential pitfalls or inappropriate techniques. Although treatment manuals have been developed to guide investigators doing group therapy research, a manual for clinicians does not exist that presents an empirically supported method of treating schizophrenic patients in therapy groups. This book remedies this situation.

The approach described in this book evolved from more than 20 years of clinical and research activities conducted by me and my colleagues. The empirical work included a controlled study of inpatient group therapy that took place in San Antonio, Texas, from 1975 to 1977, and a program of group therapy research that began in San Francisco, California, in 1978. Most of the latter work was done in association with the Department of Veterans Affairs Medical Center and the University of California in San Francisco. Therapy groups using this model also have been evaluated in Russia and England.

The initial studies took place on an acute-care inpatient psychiatric unit. As the clinical model was refined, outcome and process studies were performed. The model was extrapolated to the outpatient setting, and both short-term and long-term groups were evaluated. Important techniques were clarified, and the model was found to be replicable and teachable to a number of staff and trainees.

The primary purpose of this book is to acquaint mental health practitioners with a safe, helpful, and cost-effective method of treating schizophrenic patients using the integrative model of group therapy that evolved from the above-mentioned work. Practical guidelines and clinical vignettes are given to help the reader lead such groups in both inpatient and outpatient settings. Important theoretical and clinical issues are considered, such as treatment goals, patient selection, relevant discussion topics, and therapeutic process.

In this book, I also provide a review of the anecdotal and empirical literature dealing with the use of therapy groups with schizophrenic patients. The results from a series of outcome and process studies conducted by me and my colleagues are reviewed to provide justification for the method described in the book and to illustrate a rationale for many of the treatment techniques.

This book will be of interest to health care workers who provide services to schizophrenic patients and their families. These include staff and trainees of hospitals and clinics as well as private practitioners. The book will be of particular interest to physicians, psychologists, nurses, social workers, and other professionals who work in mental health settings. The book is relevant for students as well as experienced practitioners, for staff in state and federal hospitals as well as professionals in managed care environments and private offices, for researchers as well as clinicians, and for experienced group therapists as well as novices in this therapeutic modality.

Although this book is basically a "how-to" treatment manual, the model evolved from a program of group therapy research. Unlike many other treatment expositions, there is an empirical underpinning that gives the method validity and reliability. Theory, practice, and research are closely integrated. While integrating the best from prior models that use educative, psychodynamic, and interpersonal approaches, the model presented in this book adds new techniques and clarifies ways to formulate and deal with patient problems. References to our published research are included. Clinical vignettes from actual groups help the reader understand the model and the specific techniques that are being discussed.

The book begins with a discussion of the nature of schizophrenia in Chapter 1, including general clinical features, diagnostic considerations, biopsychosocial treatment strategies, and the role of group therapy. In Chapter 2, historical issues are reviewed, both in terms of clinical reports and research reports. Important anecdotal and empirical trends are highlighted. This is followed by a discussion of theoretical issues in Chapter 3. Three traditional approaches are described: educative, psychodynamic, and interpersonal, and the strengths and weaknesses of each are considered. The integrative approach used in this book is then considered from a theoretical point of view.

The clinical features of the treatment approach are described in the next three chapters. In Chapter 4, the focus is on the group format. Treatment goals, patient selection, co-therapy, structural issues (e.g., setting, duration and frequency of sessions, group composition and size), and the use of medications are discussed. Treatment strategies next are considered in Chapter 5. These include therapist stance, patient safety, helpful and harmful discussion topics, ways to develop these topics, coping strategies, typical progression of a topic in a session, issues related to the first and last sessions and new and departing members, pregroup orientation, and concurrent group and individual therapy. In Chapter 6, the group process is described. Topics include group dynamics, developmental stages, therapeutic factors, cultural perspectives, training and supervision, and cost-effectiveness. Case vignettes are amply used in these three chapters to illustrate important clinical issues.

In Chapter 7, the empirical work supporting this treatment model is reviewed in terms of both inpatient and outpatient studies. The findings to date are integrated in terms of outcome, process, and discussion content, and suggestions are made for future research. References to our empirical work are provided for the interested reader. This is followed by Chapter 8, a conclusions chapter that highlights the major points made in this book. Some readers may choose to read this chapter first to become oriented to the specific issues that are presented in this book. By reading the entire book in sequence, however, it is hoped that the reader will gain a thorough understanding of this integrative model and will be able to apply it in dealing with schizophrenic patients in his or her own therapy groups.

Acknowledgments

I would like to acknowledge a number of colleagues who helped me with the clinical and research work that formed the backbone of this approach: Martha Rogers, Ernie Kreth, Linda Patterson, Rick Campbell, Mary Ann Barr, Vince DiLella, Jeff Jones, Steve Dossick, Pablo Stewart, Kristi Haney, John Deri, Terry Ketter, George Fein, and A. J. Smith. I also would like to thank a number of other colleagues who supported my work along the way: John Sparks, Irwin Feinberg, I. Charles Kaufman, Craig Van Dyke, Peter Banys, Ed Merrin, Geoff Booth, Gerald Charles, Lawrence Stewart, Larry Lehmann, Dennis Farrell, Elaine Lonergan, Bob Okin, Lucy Fisher, Cindy Gyori, M. M. Kabanov, Eugene Zubkov, Steven Hirsch, and Felicity de Zulueta. Jo Ann Blackston, B. J. Kelly, and Gloria Patel provided valuable secretarial support for earlier papers, presentations, and grant proposals. Finally, I would like to thank Carolynn, Andrew, and Peter for their patience and support during the writing of this book.

CHAPTER 1

Nature of Schizophrenia

Schizophrenia is a chronic mental illness that affects the content and process of thought. Although schizophrenic patients may experience acute exacerbations that can result in hospitalization, even between such episodes their lives are affected by this disorder. Treatment usually includes attention to basic physical needs; antipsychotic medications; counseling and support; individual, group, and family therapy; recreational and occupational therapy; and a variety of social services. Because these patients often experience hallucinations and delusions, have difficulty testing reality, lead isolated lives, and have maladaptive relationships, group therapy would seem to be a natural treatment consideration. In fact, as we shall see in the next chapter, this treatment modality has been used for schizophrenic patients for more than 70 years, and an empirically derived approach for treating these patients in groups is the subject of subsequent chapters. In this chapter, I take a look at the disorder itself as well as some of the ways that group therapy might play a role in the treatment armamentarium. This overview is not meant to be exhaustive, but it introduces material that is relevant for what follows later in this book.

Symptoms and Signs of Schizophrenia

Schizophrenia is an illness that affects the way a person thinks, both at the level of what is thought about (the content of thought) and how ideas are put together (the process of thought). In terms of content, these patients may experience disorders in perception where they perceive something that is not there (hallucinations) even though their sensorium is clear. Although any sensory modality can be affected, the auditory sense is most typically involved, where the patients report hearing voices speaking to them that are perceived as being distinct from their own thoughts. In addition, schizophrenic patients may experience disorders in belief (delusions). The most common are persecutory delusions (e.g., there is an organized plot to harass them) and referential delusions (e.g., television shows have private messages specifically directed at them). Other examples include grandiose delusions (e.g., they have special powers that others do not have), thought insertion (e.g., people are placing ideas into their minds), and thought broadcasting (e.g., they can project their thoughts out to others).

When disturbances in thought content progress to the point that a patient is unable to distinguish reality from fantasy, he or she is said to be psychotic. Psychotic individuals generally cannot test reality and are prisoners of their own disordered thinking. This is to distinguish them from patients who may have similar problems in reality sense but who are not psychotic because they are able to look at their disturbances objectively and to reject or at least doubt their validity. Thus, it is possible to experience a hallucination or to have a sense that you are being followed by others while at the same time having enough reality testing ability to know that these are disturbances in your thinking and do not represent reality (Goldman 1992). Reality testing and reality sense are two important functions of the ego that are thought to be disturbed in schizophrenic patients, thus giving rise to many of the symptoms and signs of this disease. Bellak (1958) described a number of other ego functions that may be defective in these patients, including defense mechanisms, judgment, control over drives, and thought processes.

Schizophrenic patients may have serious problems in the process of their thought that lead to disorganized thinking. Most commonly, they exhibit loose associations, where one idea is followed by another idea that is poorly related to the first. At times, their thinking is vague and digressive, but it sooner or later comes back to the main point (circumstantial thinking). At other times, one idea leads to another idea that is only obliquely related, and they never return to the topic (tangential thinking). Less commonly, their thoughts are incoherently presented (word salad) or rapidly shift in a pressured manner from one idea to another (flight of ideas). These disturbances in thought may be associated with problems in affect. Some schizophrenic patients have a flat or blunted affective expression, characterized by a monotonous voice and immobile face. Others have a labile affect, where their mood state shifts abruptly, or an inappropriate affect that is not related to the content of their speech. Patients also report a variety of emotions that result from their condition, such as depression, despair, and anger. However, the hallmark of schizophrenia is a disorder of thought, not mood, and other diagnostic possibilities should be considered if the predominant symptoms and signs are in the emotional arena.

Schizophrenic patients have other problems. They usually are socially isolated and unable to relate meaningfully with others, including strangers, health care providers, employers, and family members. When they try to relate, their attempts may be maladaptively stereotyped, smothering, bizarre, distrusting, detached, or otherwise inappropriate. In addition, schizophrenic patients have a poor sense of self; a disturbance in carrying out goal-directed activity; and problems in psychomotor behavior that include catatonic stupor, rigidity or excitement, childlike silliness, agitation, and odd mannerisms. As a result, these patients have numerous social problems that are related to employment, education, finances, housing, self-care, and general quality of life.

Sometimes the symptoms of schizophrenia are divided into positive and negative categories (Africa and Schwartz 1992; American Psychiatric Association 1994). Positive symptoms are more active and represent a distortion or excess of normal functions. Examples include hallucinations, delusions, disorganized speech, and agitated behavior. They are seen early in the course of the disease, especially during acute exacerbations, and they are usually suppressed by antipsychotic medications. Negative symptoms are more passive and represent a decrease in normal functions. Examples include emotional blunting, social withdrawal, poverty of speech, and restricted behavior. They become more apparent as the disease becomes chronic, and they are usually less responsive to antipsychotic medications.

Other Features of Schizophrenia

Symptoms and signs of schizophrenia typically begin during late adolescence or early adulthood, although some forms may begin in childhood or middle age. The causes of schizophrenia are unclear; genetic, constitutional, psychodynamic, familial, and social etiologies have been implicated (Africa and Schwartz 1992; Kaplan and Sadock 1989). There usually is a prodromal phase of the disease, which is characterized by a deterioration of functioning, followed by the active phase, where psychotic symptoms are prominent, and a residual phase, which is much like the prodromal phase. Some patients experience a series of exacerbations and remissions, others a more chronic course. A return to full premorbid functioning rarely occurs, and the patients tend to deteriorate progressively or to stabilize at a lower functional and socioeconomic level.

The disease has been reported in several countries throughout the world at a prevalence rate approaching 1%. According to the American Psychiatric Association (1994), schizophrenic persons in developing nations tend to have a more acute course and a better prognosis than their counterparts in developed countries. The disease is about 10 times more common in first-degree biological relatives of schizophrenic patients than would be expected in the general population. About 10% of schizophrenic patients commit suicide, particularly men who are under age 30. It affects both sexes in roughly equal numbers, although women have a later onset, more prominent mood symptoms, and a better treatment outcome than men (Szymanski et al. 1995).

In the United States alone, some three million people will experience the pain and suffering of this disease. Millions more of their family and friends will be indirectly affected. Although less than 40% of patients admitted for psychiatric hospitalization suffer from schizophrenia (Africa and Schwartz 1992), the morbidity, chronicity, and costs of the disease make it a major health problem, particularly when one considers that it affects people from early adulthood on and prevents them from reaching their full productive potential. In a similar manner, the disorder has negative consequences for people in other countries throughout the world, and any treatment approach that can ease its impact will have major social implications.

Diagnostic Considerations

The diagnostic criteria of schizophrenia have changed throughout the years, and to some extent this has affected the reported prevalence and outcome of the disease (Hegarty et al. 1994). Currently, the two most widely used diagnostic criteria systems are the *Diagnostic and Statistical Manual of Mental Disorders* (DSM-IV) (American Psychiatric Association 1994) and the *ICD-10 Classification of Mental and Behavioural Disorders* (World Health Organization 1992). Table 1–1 lists some of the main features of schizophrenia that are outlined in DSM-IV. For a complete description of the criteria, the reader is referred to DSM-IV.

As can be seen from Table 1–1, two or more characteristic symptoms of the disease need to be present for at least 1 month, although some signs of schizophrenia have to be present for at least 6 months. There also needs to be evidence of social or occupational dysfunction since the disturbance began, and functioning should be below the level achieved prior to the onset. Finally, conditions described in DSM-IV that might be confused with this disease should be excluded.

A number of subtypes of schizophrenia are recognized, and their key characteristics are summarized in Table 1–2. All must meet the basic criteria for schizophrenia, but they differ in terms of predominant symptomatology at the time of evaluation. It is useful to distinguish these different subtypes because of prognostic and treatment implications. For example, paranoid schizo-

Table 1–1. Diagnostic criteria for schizophrenia

Two or more of the following symptoms are present for at least 1 month: delusions, hallucinations, disorganized speech, disorganized or catatonic behavior, negative symptoms.

Continuous signs of the disturbance for at least 6 months.

Social or occupational dysfunction since the onset of the disturbance.

The following are excluded: schizoaffective disorder, mood disorder, physiological effects of substance use or medical condition, simple continuation of pervasive developmental disorder.

Note. Adapted from DSM-IV.

phrenia tends to occur later in life and to be less severe than the other subtypes, whereas the disorganized subtype tends to occur earliest, have an insidious and continuous course, and be most severe (American Psychiatric Association 1994). The main feature of the paranoid subtype is a preoccupation with delusions or frequent auditory hallucinations. Other symptoms of schizophrenia (e.g., disorganized speech, disorganized or catatonic behavior, negative symptoms) are absent or at least not prominent. In contrast, the disorganized subtype must have disorganized speech and behavior as well as flat or inappropriate affect. Delusions, hallucinations, and catatonia are not present or are fragmentary. The essential feature of the catatonic subtype is a marked psychomotor disturbance, regardless of the presence of other symptoms of schizophrenia. The diagnosis is made if the clinical picture is dominated by at least two of the following: catalepsy or stupor, excessive purposeless motor activity, extreme negativism or mutism, peculiar voluntary movements (e.g., pos-

Table 1–2. Subtypes of schizophrenia

Subtype	Key characteristics
Paranoid	Delusions or frequent auditory hallucinations
	No other symptoms of schizophrenia
Disorganized	Disorganized speech and behavior
	Flat or inappropriate affect
Catatonic	At least two examples of psychomotor disturbance (e.g., immobility, excessive activity, negativism or mutism, peculiar voluntary movements, echolalia, or echopraxia)
Undifferentiated	Two or more symptoms of schizophrenia
	Absence of criteria for other subtypes
Residual	Absence of prominent positive symptoms of schizophrenia
	Continuous evidence of the disturbance (e.g., negative symptoms, attenuated positive symptoms)

Note. Adapted from DSM-IV.

turing, stereotypy, mannerisms, grimacing), and echolalia (repetition of another person's speech) or echopraxia (repetition of another person's movements). In the undifferentiated subtype, there are at least two or more characteristic symptoms of schizophrenia, but the criteria for the paranoid, disorganized, and catatonic subtypes are not met. Finally, in the residual subtype, there is a history of at least one episode of schizophrenia and continuing evidence of the disturbance. For example, there may be negative symptoms or two or more positive symptoms that are attenuated (e.g., unusual but nondelusional beliefs, odd perceptual experiences). However, there are no prominent delusions, hallucinations, disorganized speech, or disorganized or catatonic behaviors.

There are a number of related psychiatric conditions that are shown in Chapter 4 to be amenable to treatment in groups involving schizophrenic patients. These are listed in Table 1–3, along with some key characteristics. It should be noted that for all of these conditions, the characteristics should not be due to the

Table 1–3. Conditions related to schizophrenia

Condition	Key characteristics
Schizophreniform disorder	Criteria similar to schizophrenia, but disturbance lasts from 1 to 6 months.
	Social or occupational dysfunction is not required.
Schizoaffective disorder	An uninterrupted period of illness where a major depressive, manic, or mixed episode coexists for a substantial period of time with symptoms of schizophrenia.
	During this same period of illness, delusions or hallucinations exist for at least 2 weeks in the absence of mood symptoms.
Delusional disorder	Nonbizarre delusions are present for at least 1 month without a prominent mood episode or a history of symptoms typical of schizophrenia.
	Functioning is not markedly impaired, and behavior is not obviously bizarre.

Note. Adapted from DSM-IV.

physiological effects of substance use or to some other medical condition. Schizophreniform disorder is similar to schizophrenia, but the duration of the disturbance is from 1 to 6 months. In addition, there is no requirement for social or occupational dysfunction to be present. In schizoaffective disorder, there needs to be a long period of time where symptoms of schizophrenia and symptoms of a mood episode coexist. However, this period needs to be preceded or followed by at least 2 weeks of delusions or hallucinations without evidence of mood symptoms. Finally, in a delusional disorder, nonbizarre delusions have to be present for at least 1 month in the absence of a prominent mood episode or other symptoms that are typical of schizophrenia. In addition, functioning is not markedly impaired, and behavior is not obviously strange or bizarre.

Treatment Issues

Schizophrenia is a disorder with biological, psychological, and social causes and effects (Africa and Schwartz 1992; Kaplan and Sadock 1989). Consequently, in developing a treatment plan for patients with this disease, biomedical as well as psychosocial approaches need to be considered. This is in keeping with the biopsychosocial perspective that provides the basic framework for treatment in most psychiatric disorders (Engel 1980).

Biomedical considerations include careful attention to the physical and nutritional status of schizophrenic patients, many of whom are in poor health and have problems with self-care. In addition, antipsychotic medications are useful in reducing symptoms, allowing more patients to be treated in the community, decreasing relapse and rehospitalization rates, and generally improving outcome. Unfortunately, these potent drugs also produce acute side effects, such as sedation, hypotension, extrapyramidal symptoms, dystonia, anticholinergic effects, and the potentially dangerous neuroleptic malignant syndrome. More chronically, some patients develop tardive dyskinesia. Consequently, many patients refuse to take their medications on a regular basis when they are prescribed in pill form, and they then become candidates for the long-acting injectable (depot) form.

Most patients require antipsychotic medications during much of their lives, and these drugs are viewed by some clinicians as the major treatment intervention. However, not all schizophrenic patients achieve optimal stability with medications alone, and some patients refuse to take them or develop debilitating side effects, such as tardive dyskinesia, that limit their use. Consequently, psychosocial approaches also are necessary to maximize the treatment benefits for these patients.

Psychosocial interventions include long-term counseling and support; individual, group, and family therapy; recreational and occupational therapy; and social services related to basic areas of functioning, such as employment, education, finances, housing, and self-care. These psychosocial strategies are not only supportive and educational, but they can also help patients improve their relationships with others and cope with psychotic experiences (Breier and Strauss 1983; Cohen and Berk 1985; Corrigan and Storzbach 1993; Dobson et al. 1995; Falloon and Talbot 1981; Kanas and Barr 1984). Psychosocial interventions can be delivered in both inpatient and outpatient settings in treatment programs ranging from hospital wards and day treatment centers to clinicians' offices and mental health clinics.

A complete biopsychosocial treatment approach enhances compliance and improves prognosis. This is important in a disorder where historically not even half of the patients have shown substantial clinical improvement after long-term follow-up (Hegarty et al. 1994). A number of other factors improve prognosis, including good premorbid adjustment; acute onset, especially if there are precipitating events; later age at onset; associated mood disturbance; good interepisode functioning; and normal neurological status (American Psychiatric Association 1994).

Role of Group Therapy in Schizophrenia

According to the biopsychosocial perspective, group therapy would be included as one of the psychosocial treatment approaches. In group therapy, changes occur in patients as a result of their interactions with other patients and at least one trained therapist in a group setting. Therapeutic results include the relief of symptoms and the resolution of intrapsychic and interpersonal problems (Kanas 1992). This modality of treatment has been used for a variety of psychiatric conditions in both inpatient and outpatient settings, and it generally has been shown to be helpful as well as cost effective.

Given the characteristics of schizophrenia, group therapy would seem to an appropriate treatment option. These patients suffer from a variety of symptoms that are quite disturbing and debilitating, such as delusions, hallucinations, disorganized speech, disorganized or catatonic behavior, and a number of negative symptoms. Any treatment approach that helps them learn to cope with these symptoms could go a long way toward relieving their suffering. In addition, they also experience intrapsychic distress when not actively psychotic during the prodromal and residual periods. A group experience could give them support and help them gain an understanding of ways to reduce stress, relieve psychic tension, and test reality should they find themselves slipping back into a more active state. Finally, schizophrenic patients tend to be isolative people who relate poorly with others. Because group therapy is essentially an interpersonal treatment modality, having a forum to talk about relationship issues with people who have similar problems could be very enlightening. In addition, in the process of interacting with other group members, the patients are practicing social skills that could be extrapolated to interpersonal situations outside of the sessions. Consequently, interpersonal problems could be addressed in two ways: through the discussions and through the process of the group experience itself.

Thus, there are several reasons why group therapy might be useful for schizophrenic patients. Is it, in fact, useful? And if so, what kind of approach works best? Are there any approaches that are harmful? I begin to answer these questions in the next chapter.

References

Africa B, Schwartz SR: Schizophrenic disorders, in Review of General Psychiatry, 3rd Edition. Edited by Goldman HH. Norwalk, CT, Appleton & Lange, 1992, pp 198–214

American Psychiatric Association: Schizophrenia and other psychotic disorders, in Diagnostic and Statistical Manual of Mental Disorders, 4th Edition. Washington, DC, American Psychiatric Association, 1994, pp 273–315

Bellak L (ed): Schizophrenia: A Review of the Syndrome. New York, Logos Press, 1958

Breier A, Strauss JS: Self-control in psychotic disorders. Arch Gen Psychiatry 40:1141–1145, 1983

Cohen CI, Berk LA: Personal coping styles of schizophrenic outpatients. Hosp Community Psychiatry 36:407–410, 1985

Corrigan PW, Storzbach DM: Behavioral interventions for alleviating psychotic symptoms. Hosp Community Psychiatry 44:341–347, 1993

Dobson DJG, McDougall G, Busheikin J, et al: Effects of social skills training and social milieu treatment on symptoms of schizophrenia. Psychiatric Services 46:376–380, 1995

Engel GL: The clinical application of the biopsychosocial model. Am J Psychiatry 137:535–544, 1980

Falloon IRH, Talbot RE: Persistent auditory hallucinations: coping mechanisms and implications for management. Psychol Med 11:329–339, 1981

Goldman HH (ed): Review of General Psychiatry, 3rd Edition. Norwalk, CT, Appleton & Lange, 1992

Hegarty JD, Baldessarini RJ, Tohen M, et al: One hundred years of schizophrenia: a meta-analysis of the outcome literature. Am J Psychiatry 151:1409–1416, 1994

Kanas N: Group psychotherapy, in Review of General Psychiatry, 3rd Edition. Edited by Goldman HH. Norwalk, CT, Appleton & Lange, 1992, pp 417–423

Kanas N, Barr MA: Self-control of psychotic productions in schizophrenics. Arch Gen Psychiatry 41:919–920, 1984

Kaplan HI, Sadock BJ (eds): Comprehensive Textbook of Psychiatry, 5th Edition. Baltimore, MD, Williams & Wilkins, 1989

Szymanski S, Lieberman JA, Alvir JM, et al: Gender differences in onset of illness, treatment response, course, and biological indexes in first-episode schizophrenic patients. Am J Psychiatry 152:698–703, 1995

World Health Organization: The ICD-10 Classification of Mental and Behavioural Disorders. Geneva, Switzerland, World Health Organization, 1992

CHAPTER 2

Historical Issues

Schizophrenic patients have been treated in therapy groups for more than 70 years. Published clinical reports on this approach have been descriptive in nature, and the authors have been optimistic in discussing the benefits of group therapy for psychotic patients. In a more objective manner, controlled studies also have advocated the use of group therapy for schizophrenic patients. Particularly since the 1950s, when phenothiazines began to be used in the clinical setting, this empirical work has demonstrated that group therapy is a useful adjunct to antipsychotic medications for these patients and in many cases is superior to individual therapy. This anecdotal and empirical work is reviewed in this chapter.

Clinical Reports

Because the clinical reports have spanned such a long period of time, the methods and settings have varied a great deal. A number of factors have contributed to this variation, including changing preferences in psychotherapeutic technique, differing philosophies regarding mental health care delivery, and the advent of antipsychotic medications (Engel 1980; Hegarty et al. 1994). Schizophrenic patients have been treated in settings ranging from chronic long-term state institutions to acute-care rapid discharge units in general hospitals, and from comprehensive day treatment centers to outpatient clinics and private offices. In addition, the diagnostic system of classifying the disorder has varied, from the early dementia praecox days to the diagnoses that were based on psychodynamic formulations and finally to the more descriptive and phenomenologically oriented classification systems that we use today (American Psychiatric Association 1994; World Health Organization 1992). For all these reasons, it may be difficult to compare one report with another. Taken together, however, they present a fascinating picture of the ways in which therapists have treated schizophrenic patients in groups, and they set the stage for the theoretical issues that are discussed in Chapter 3.

Early History

The first person to describe the use of group techniques to treat schizophrenic patients was Lazell (1921). He believed that the goals of treatment included educating patients about facets of the illness as well as about basic psychic development, directing instinctive demands into normal channels, and improving social adjustment. His approach utilized psychodynamic concepts and educational techniques, generally presented in a lecture format. Topics included the fear of death, explanations of hallucinations and delusions, self-love, inferiority and its causes, and various sexual themes. He argued for a homogeneous approach: "Only such patients as presented the same fundamental problem and were solving their difficulties in the same manner should be included in the same group" (p. 170). He listed several advantages to his group method: patients became more socialized, they feared the therapist less, previously inaccessible patients were able to hear and retain much of the material, they reacted positively and discussed the lectures with each other after the sessions, and the negative effects of institutionalization were countered. Although some patients temporarily became worse by being confronted with the material, in the long run Lazell believed his method to be constructive. He took a proactive role regarding the treatment of patients with dementia praecox (i.e., schizophrenia):

> Institutions for the insane now largely devoted to custodial care, hydrotherapy, etc., should be changed into institutions for the instruction of these patients. . . . Society owes it to these patients that they be not allowed to stagnate in mental inactivity, and that large numbers could by this method be raised to a sufficiently

high level to be of economic value to the community or return
to active life, even if on a lower plane. (p. 179)

Marsh (1933) subsequently described a treatment program at
Worcester State Hospital in Massachusetts wherein psychotic patients attended lectures and a variety of therapeutic group activities. These included presentations of inspirational music, talks on
current events, occupational therapy, and discussion groups that
included topics related to the hospital and to the symptoms and
progress of the patients. The program also included group activities for the staff, the students, the relatives of the patients, and the
community at large. He saw the mental hospital as "preeminently
an educational-social-industrial community" (p. 416). He stated
that "mental patients are susceptible to the group approach"
(p. 415), and he believed that "physicians who study psychiatry
should have a wide social training and be able to handle patients
in groups" (p. 415).

Growth of Psychoanalytic Approaches

Although a number of writers began experimenting with the use
of psychoanalytic group techniques, they primarily treated
nonpsychotic patients (Burrow 1927; Wender 1936). An exception
was Schilder (1939), who treated neurotic and psychotic patients
together in outpatient groups meeting once or twice a week. He
utilized a number of classical psychoanalytic principles and techniques, including discussions of early infantile material and sexual
development, dream analysis, insight, free association, the explo-
ration of the unconscious, and transference interpretations. Schilder saw the group as being valuable for helping "the patients
realize with astonishment that the thoughts which have seemed
to isolate them are common to all of them" (p. 91). In reviewing
the outcome of 49 patients treated in his group, he classified 5 as
being schizophrenic. Of these, he thought that 3 were unchanged,
1 showed some improvement, and 1 recovered completely.

After World War II, Semrad (1948) and his colleagues at the
Boston State Hospital began describing their use of psychoanalytic techniques to treat psychotic patients in groups. Semrad
viewed the groups as helping the patients orient their attitudes
to understand personal problems better and to participate more

spontaneously in life. He saw the therapist as a catalyst who takes his or her cues from the group members and "makes comments, listens, smiles and does whatever seems appropriate to keep up a free and easy conversation" (p. 109). Catharsis and group unity were seen as helpful therapeutic factors, and patient-to-patient advice regarding personal problems was welcomed. He described the work of the group as follows: "Patients introspect, mutually criticize and work through these emotional problems. After this comes their attempt to deal with more reality issues, important in their future lives" (p. 109).

In a follow-up paper by Standish and Semrad (1951), the groups were described as meeting for 1 hour two or three times a week. Although they could accommodate a maximum of 15 patients, 10 or 11 were preferable. Four stages of group development over time were recognized and characterized by 1) revelations of mutual hostility toward the hospital, which lead to group unity; 2) expressions of anxiety-laden psychotic material; 3) introspection and working through of emotional problems; and 4) issues of termination (e.g., discussing future plans after discharge). These authors were among the first to elucidate clearly the value of cohesion in groups of psychotic patients:

> A "poor" group we feel is one with much disorganization and chaos and great indirectness of language. . . . A "good" group on the other hand is a group in which there is a general feeling of cohesion or working together with attentiveness on the part of individual members and participation and interaction of at least a few of the members. (p. 147)

Group resistance was seen to arise from the current relationship between the patients and the therapist, and it was characterized by hostile acts, accentuated defenses, regression, and blocks in the discussion. Overall, the authors believed that their group approach was helpful, and they reported on the results of a survey of 165 patients (52% schizophrenic) who were treated in 12 separate groups that showed that about twice as many acute than chronic patients were improved enough to be sent home on a trial visit.

In 1947, psychiatrists at the Brooklyn State Hospital in New York began to treat schizophrenic patients in inpatient and outpatient therapy groups. The groups met at weekly intervals, usually for 90 minutes, and they used a psychoanalytic orientation (Lawton 1951; Pinney 1956). The therapists generally were passive and allowed the patients to analyze their own problems. At times, they made transference interpretations. The patients were encouraged to help one another gain insight into deep-seated conflicts. Topics that were frequently discussed included overprotective parents, guilt feelings, sexual problems, and emotional unrest. Although the groups were seen as useful, some members became dangerously hostile toward one another, and paranoid patients sometimes incorporated the therapist's comments into their delusional system and had to be removed from the group.

The 1950s and 1960s

Although psychoanalytic groups continued to be used for schizophrenic patients, other approaches were advocated in the 1950s and 1960s. Harking back to the time of Lazell (1921) and Marsh (1933), Klapman (1950, 1951) described a didactic group approach that involved lectures and outside homework assignments. In addition, he strongly advocated the use of a textbook. Besides the obvious educational advantages, the textbook had psychological benefits as well: "The text performs the function of stimulus, calling forth patients' responses and reactions, often stimulating the production of deeper material and associated abreaction" (Klapman 1950, p. 41). His method encouraged the members to interact and discuss topics of interest, and he allowed digressions that he believed were worthwhile. Patients participating in 3 months of his groups showed improvements on the Bell Adjustment Inventory and the Rorschach (Klapman 1951).

Frank (1955) took a different point of view in discussing group therapy with hospitalized patients, many of whom were schizophrenic. He stated that

> The object of psychotherapy is to supply new interpersonal influences which help the patient resolve his conflicts, develop a more accurate picture of himself in relation to others, and so become able to behave more fittingly towards them. As the patient begins to experience some successes in his dealings with others, this reinforces the new ways of behaving; and so, if all goes well, the maladaptive patterns are progressively weakened and the more successful ones strengthened. (p. 2)

Given this strong interpersonal orientation, Frank saw group therapy as a valuable treatment modality. He stated that

> The task of a therapeutic group activity is an important means of fostering a sense of belongingness among the members. It does this by giving them a common focus which encourages them to relate to each other and supplying a vehicle for them to do so. (p. 5)

He termed this sense of belongingness "group cohesiveness," and he viewed this as a major therapeutic factor that should be strongly encouraged by the therapist. This could be done by actively keeping the group on task, facilitating patient communication, and encouraging productive interactions. He viewed group therapy with hospitalized patients as needing to keep tension "within bounds," and he saw schizophrenic patients as being particularly vulnerable to close emotional contact. Thus, therapists should guard against producing a group environment that was too stimulating, and he believed that a nondirective approach with an emphasis on insight could create intolerable anxiety in psychotic patients that might actually impede progress.

Beard et al. (1958) described the use of activity group therapy with chronically regressed hospitalized schizophrenic patients. The groups consisted of four to five members, and the therapist worked hard to establish a supportive relationship with each patient even before he or she began participating. Activities ranged from reading to solving arithmetic problems on a blackboard to playing kick the ball. Although there was little patient-to-patient interaction during the initial stages of a group, this gradually increased as continuing members began to help new arrivals. The authors believed that their approach was successful in decreasing social isolation, improving the chances for discharge, and lowering the rehospitalization rates of the members who participated.

Slavson (1961) took the position that "psychotherapy in which unconscious drives and affect-laden memories and experiences are uncovered is most often not suitable for borderline, latent, or active schizophrenic patients" (p. 27). He pointed out that because the ego of these patients is weak and their defenses are fragile, insight-oriented group therapy may be deleterious and dangerous. Instead, he advocated supportive, reality-oriented

discussions for schizophrenic patients. As patients went into re-
mission, he speculated that they benefited from "their growing
relatedness as a result of the comfort, intimacy, and sharing that
occur in a small group" (p. 27).

In contrast, Alikakos (1965) advocated the use of analytical,
insight-oriented group therapy for posthospitalized schizophrenic patients. He believed that the transference reactions were
less intense than in individual therapy, and the patients had a
more comfortable relationship with the therapist. His long-term
approach included support, enhanced reality testing, and graded
socializing experiences. These latter characteristics may have attenuated the ego-disruptive qualities of uncovering techniques
that so worried Slavson (1961).

Finally, Horowitz and Weisberg (1966) described the value of
using directive techniques to structure productively the group
environment in their inpatient therapy groups for schizophrenic
patients. They envisioned "three basic goals of treatment: 1) establishing and maintaining group cohesiveness; 2) establishing
meaningful group and individual patient participation; and
3) discouraging self-impairing responses and behavior in patients" (p. 43). To achieve these goals, they advocated techniques
that employed "active, directive, even charismatic and manipu-
lative measures to ameliorate the estrangement, confusions, and
anxiety of acute psychosis" (p. 48). Some of these techniques included paraphrasing tangential comments made by the patients
into coherent statements, isolating agitated or dominant members from the discussion, making interim or closing summaries,
applying group pressure to encourage the participation of withdrawn patients, and establishing modest yet achievable goals for
the members. At times, nonverbal techniques were used that involved the therapist's posture, direction of gaze, facial expression,
and vocal modulation. Although the authors worried that some
of their techniques were authoritarian and encouraged dependency, they admitted that they seemed to work when used flex-
ibly in an atmosphere of understanding.

Recent History

During the past 20 years, a number of papers have been published
describing ways to treat schizophrenic patients in therapy groups.

Most of these are extensions of the approaches discussed earlier; for this reason, they are only summarized here. Others are mentioned because they present a new technique or principle that the interested reader may wish to pursue. Current representative examples of the major theoretical models are discussed at length in Chapter 3.

Some authors have used educative approaches that focus on didactic issues. Most of these consist of presentations or lectures that involve aspects of the members' illness (e.g., symptoms or course), and these are followed by group discussions (Fenn and Dinaburg 1981; Maxmen 1978; Plante et al. 1988). These discussions not only clarify some of the didactic issues, but they also allow the members to express their feelings and interact with one another, which can be quite helpful for isolated schizophrenic patients.

A more specialized educative approach employs groups that focus on social skills training (Dobson et al. 1995; Douglas and Mueser 1990; Hierholzer and Liberman 1986), and these may be used as part of a complete rehabilitation program that includes individual counseling and independent living services. Although the groups aim at improving the social skills of the patients, the basic style is educative: "Training sessions resemble a classroom environment more than a traditional therapy setting, with therapists utilizing visual aids (e.g., posters listing the skills) and teaching skills in a systematic format" (Douglas and Mueser 1990, p. 528). These groups use techniques that include problem identification, the attainment of clearly defined goals, role-playing, and homework assignments between sessions. They are more useful for chronic patients in long-term settings than for acutely disturbed patients in short-term settings (Dobson et al. 1995; Geczy and Sultenfuss 1995).

Other authors have expanded the psychodynamic approach to address current psychoanalytic concepts as they apply to therapy groups with schizophrenic patients. Examples of these concepts have been object relations theory (Kibel 1981, 1987, 1991; Milders 1994; Takahashi and Washington 1991) and self psychology (Josephs and Juman 1985). Other psychodynamic offshoots have included group analysis (Chazan 1993; Sandison 1991, 1994), group-as-a-whole principles (Malawista and Malawista 1988), and ideas stemming from the theories of Wilfred Bion (Johnson et al. 1986; Kapur 1993). Mindful of the dangers of intense anxiety and strong affect on the fragile egos of psychotic patients, some therapists have incorporated techniques to minimize the potential problems of an insight-oriented, uncovering approach. Examples of these techniques have been the liberal use of supportive comments and an active, directive style that structures the group process in ways that help advance the group goals.

The interpersonal approach also has been represented (Kahn 1984; Yalom 1983; Yehoshua et al. 1985). As before, the focus has been on improving the ability of schizophrenic patients to relate better with other people and to become less isolative in their daily lives. The group has been viewed as a way for the members to practice and improve their interactive skills. In addition, many interpersonally oriented therapists have placed great emphasis on group cohesion and on making comments involving the interactions between the members during the group sessions. Particularly for more regressed schizophrenic patients, formal interpersonal exercises have been used to break the ice and to encourage the patients to relate better with each other.

More specialized approaches also have been advocated. Examples have included groups utilizing Gestalt concepts (Serok et al. 1984) and encounter techniques (Sandison 1975); groups that focus on open discussion and affect expression, but which also incorporate special modifications for psychotic patients (Gruber 1978; Klein 1977); groups using videotapes that are later played back to the patients for discussion (Gunn 1978); patient-led groups that are observed by staff who later discuss what they saw in front of the group members (Gould et al. 1975); medication groups (Gordon et al. 1994); supportive drop-in groups that depend on institutional transference and do not require regular attendance by the members (Misunis et al. 1990); groups using cognitive deficits (Erickson 1986) or the ability to relate interpersonally (Leopold 1976) as criteria to determine membership; and flexible-boundaried groups that allow patients to determine the frequency of their attendance (McIntosh et al. 1991).

Trends: Clinical Reports

A number of trends were discerned from the clinical literature. Despite being conducted in a variety of settings for more than

70 years, the reports generally were positive and even enthusiastic. The patients did well, as determined by clinical impression and in some cases by formal surveys. Many of the patients were very regressed and institutionalized, and they were treated in groups in the era before phenothiazines. These facts made the claims by the authors even more remarkable. There seemed to be three major orientations characterizing most of the groups: educative, psychodynamic, and interpersonal. Approaches using educational techniques were written about earliest. The psychodynamic approach followed and seemed to parallel the increasing popularity of psychoanalysis. However, some authors suggested that this orientation in its pure form could be too stressful for schizophrenic patients, and they began to include support and structure in their techniques. Finally, the interpersonal approach was introduced as therapists began to appreciate the value of fostering group cohesion and making comments on group member interactions. These three traditional orientations continue to be used today, sometimes in updated versions, as is described in Chapter 3. However, many current therapy groups for schizophrenic patients are more eclectic and use mixtures of these approaches. In addition, specialized techniques (e.g., videotape playback, flexible drop-in groups) have been added to the armamentarium.

Research Reports

To evaluate the effectiveness of therapy groups for schizophrenic patients more objectively, I made a literature review of controlled studies dating back to the time that antipsychotic medications began to be used in the clinical setting. Because these drugs have such a profound beneficial effect on psychotic patients, and because they are generally considered to be a major treatment modality for schizophrenia (Africa and Schwartz 1992; Kaplan and Sadock 1989), I could not envision using group therapy with this disorder in any modern program where these drugs were not readily available. Consequently, in my survey, all of the studies evaluated group therapy in the context of concomitant antipsychotic medications.

The review encompassed more than 40 years, from 1950 to 1991, and it was an extension of an earlier survey I conducted in the mid-1980s (Kanas 1986a). Interestingly, the extension added only 3 additional studies (all outpatient) to the original 43. To be included in the review, the studies had to meet the following criteria: 1) compare at least one group therapy condition with a comparable control condition, such as free time on the ward, individual therapy, or some other group activity; 2) indicate clearly that more than half of the people being evaluated were schizophrenic or statistically partial out the effects of the group on schizophrenic patients; 3) include at least one major measure of outcome that addressed the effectiveness of group therapy; and 4) state the duration of treatment in terms of number of sessions or some unit of time (e.g., weeks or months). A total of 46 studies met these criteria; 33 involved inpatient groups, and 13 involved outpatient groups.

Because the studies spanned such a long period of time, they varied in terms of the diagnostic criteria used. For example, a few of the earlier reports used the first edition of the DSM (American Psychiatric Association 1952), whereas some of the later ones used DSM-II (American Psychiatric Association 1968), DSM-III (American Psychiatric Association 1980), or DSM-III-R (American Psychiatric Association 1987). Others employed a different classification system or did not specify what criteria they used in establishing the diagnosis of schizophrenia. In addition, the treatment settings varied, although all of the programs included antipsychotic medications. Specific group therapy techniques were described with varying degrees of completeness, but it usually was easy to determine the main clinical orientation of the groups.

Methodologically, the outcome measures that were used differed among the studies, from discharge and rehospitalization rates to measures of symptoms and improved social skills. Also, the statistical metrics varied greatly and, in some cases, were reported incompletely. This made it difficult to use meta-analytic techniques (Kanas 1986a, 1986b). However, in all cases, significance levels between the experimental and control conditions were reported or could be calculated from the data, and this became the basis of my analysis. Each study was taken as a unit and was categorized in terms of whether it supported the conclusion that group therapy was significantly better than, equal to, or significantly worse than the no-group control condition.

The studies were evaluated in terms of whether they were

inpatient or outpatient. They also were categorized in terms of the duration of the groups: long-term (37+ sessions), intermediate-term (18–36 sessions), and short-term (17 or fewer sessions). For the inpatient studies, these session numbers generally corresponded to an average of greater than 3 months, 6 weeks to 3 months, and less than 6 weeks, respectively. Things were a bit more confusing for the outpatient setting, where there was a broader range in terms of duration (9–220 sessions) and frequency (weekly to monthly). Although more than half of the groups met for fewer than 37 sessions (placing them in the short-to-intermediate range), several of these were held on an infrequent basis (e.g., monthly), and so they continued for more than 3 months, which would be considered long-term. To be consistent with the inpatient groups, I used the number of sessions rather than time passed as the best indication of treatment duration for the outpatient groups.

I also was interested in evaluating the relative effectiveness of the clinical orientation of the groups. In an earlier study, I had concluded that an insight-oriented group therapy approach might be harmful for schizophrenic patients (Kanas et al. 1980), and I was interested in examining what others had found. Consequently, all of the 57 therapy groups that were evaluated in the 46 studies were placed into one of three clinical categories, which are summarized in Table 2–1. Each group that represented a specific category then was classified as to whether it was significantly better than, equal to, or significantly worse than its corresponding no-group control condition. This allowed me to evaluate the overall advantages of the three clinical approaches.

Effectiveness of Group Therapy With Schizophrenic Patients

Table 2–2 summarizes the effectiveness of group therapy with schizophrenic patients in terms of the number of studies that indicated that this modality of treatment was significantly better than, equal to, or significantly worse than the no-group control condition. As can be seen, 67% of the inpatient studies found that group therapy was significantly better than the no-group condition. Interestingly, two of the studies (Kanas et al. 1980; Pattison et al. 1967) concluded that patients in the group condition became

Table 2–1. Clinical categories of therapy groups in the
survey of controlled studies

Therapy group	Goal	Examples of techniques
Insight oriented	Improve self-understanding through the exploration of developmental and psychodynamic issues	Uncovering, transference interpretations
Interaction oriented	Improve the patients' abilities to relate better with others	Discussions of interpersonal problems and solutions, comments on member interactions during the sessions
Other/ unspecified	Neither of the above, or unclear which techniques predominated	Gestalt, psychoeducational, behavioral, activity oriented

Table 2–2. Effectiveness of group therapy for schizophrenic
patients: number and percentage of controlled studies

Comparison	Inpatient		Outpatient		Total	
	N	%	N	%	N	%
Group therapy significantly *better* than no group therapy	22	67	10	77	32	70
No difference between group therapy and no group therapy	9	27	3	23	12	26
Group therapy significantly *worse* than no group therapy	2	6	0	0	2	4
Total	33	100	13	100	46	100

significantly worse than those in the no-group condition, thus demonstrating that any effective treatment can be potentially harmful as well as helpful. There was a nonsignificant trend in favor of longer-term groups: 79% of the long-term studies supported group therapy over the no-group condition, as compared with 60% and 56% of the intermediate- and short-term studies, respectively (Kanas 1986a).

In the outpatient setting, 77% of the studies favored the group therapy condition over the control condition. Group therapy was found to be at least as effective or more effective than individual therapy in the four studies where this comparison was made. There did not seem to be a relationship between the number of sessions and effectiveness (possibly because so many of the 13 studies were positive). In reviewing the group descriptions, the outpatient groups met less frequently, had more members, and were more homogeneous in terms of diagnosis than their inpatient counterparts. The patients seemed to value their experience, and the attendance rates were high, sometimes reaching 95% or greater (Alden et al. 1979; Donlon et al. 1973).

Overall, 70% of the studies were in favor of group therapy. The success rate did not differ greatly between inpatient groups (particularly those that were long-term) and outpatient groups. Thus, this literature review generally supported the effectiveness of group therapy for schizophrenic patients, when it was used in conjunction with antipsychotic medications.

Influence of Clinical Orientation

Table 2–3 shows the number of groups that were judged to be significantly better than their corresponding no-group control condition in terms of whether the predominant clinical approach of each group was insight oriented, interaction oriented, or other/unspecified (see Table 2–1 for operational definitions). In the inpatient setting, only 30% of the insight groups were significantly better versus 76% of the interaction groups and 53% of the other/unspecified category. The difference in proportion between insight and interaction categories was significant using Fisher's exact test. There was a similar but nonsignificant trend for outpatient groups. Overall, fewer insight-oriented groups were found to be superior to their control groups (33%) than interaction-oriented groups (78%) or other/unspecified groups (59%). Again, the difference between insight and interaction categories was significant. Three of the studies directly compared insight with interaction groups. One of these studies (Coons 1957) found the interaction approach to be significantly better, whereas two others (Roback 1972; Semon and Goldstein 1957) found no difference. Three additional studies concluded that their insight-oriented groups produced worse results than other groups or a no-group control condition (Kanas et al. 1980; MacDonald et al. 1964; Pattison et al. 1967). It should be noted that all of these studies took place on inpatient units. Nevertheless, these findings are in keeping with other reports that suggest that an insight-oriented, uncovering treatment approach may be harmful for schizophrenic patients (Drake and Sederer 1986; Geczy and Sultenfuss 1995; Strassberg et al. 1975; Weiner 1984).

Trends: Research Reports

A number of trends emerged from the research literature. Group therapy was effective for schizophrenic patients in both inpatient and outpatient settings. Of the studies that were reviewed, 70% found this modality of treatment to be significantly better than a

Table 2–3. Influence of clinical category on group therapy effectiveness for schizophrenic patients, controlled studies: proportion and percentage of groups that were significantly better than corresponding no-group control condition

Setting	Insight category		Interaction category		Other/ unspecified	
	Proportion	%	Proportion	%	Proportion	%
Inpatient	3/10	30[*]	13/17	76[*]	9/17	53
Outpatient	1/2	50	5/6	83	4/5	80
Total	4/12	33[**]	18/23	78[**]	13/22	59

[*]P < .0402, two-tailed, Fisher's exact test.
[**]P < .0135, two-tailed, Fisher's exact test.

no-group therapy control condition, and group therapy was found to be as effective or more effective than individual therapy for schizophrenic patients in the outpatient studies that included this comparison. There was a tendency for long-term inpatient groups to be more beneficial than short- and intermediate-term groups. Insight-oriented approaches that emphasized uncovering and psychodynamic issues were significantly less effective for schizophrenic patients than interaction-oriented approaches that focused on relationships and interpersonal problems. This was especially true in the inpatient setting. Furthermore, insight-oriented techniques were harmful for some inpatient schizophrenic patients in groups. These patients were better off having free time on the ward than engaging in a treatment modality that might have been too stimulating for their fragile egos.

References

Africa B, Schwartz SR: Schizophrenic disorders, in Review of General Psychiatry, 3rd Edition. Edited by Goldman HH. Norwalk, CT, Appleton & Lange, 1992, pp 198–214

Alden AR, Weddington WW Jr, Jacobson C, et al: Group aftercare for chronic schizophrenia. J Clin Psychiatry 40:6–12, 1979

Alikakos LC: Analytical group treatment of the post-hospital schizophrenic. Int J Group Psychother 15:492–504, 1965

American Psychiatric Association: Diagnostic and Statistical Manual: Mental Disorders. Washington, DC, American Psychiatric Association, 1952

American Psychiatric Association: Diagnostic and Statistical Manual of Mental Disorders, 2nd Edition. Washington, DC, American Psychiatric Association, 1968

American Psychiatric Association: Diagnostic and Statistical Manual of Mental Disorders, 3rd Edition. Washington, DC, American Psychiatric Association, 1980

American Psychiatric Association: Diagnostic and Statistical Manual of Mental Disorders, 3rd Edition, Revised. Washington, DC, American Psychiatric Association, 1987

American Psychiatric Association: Diagnostic and Statistical Manual of Mental Disorders, 4th Edition. Washington, DC, American Psychiatric Association, 1994

Beard JH, Goertzel V, Pearce AJ: The effectiveness of activity group therapy with chronically regressed adult schizophrenics. Int J Group Psychother 8:123–136, 1958

Burrow T: The group method of analysis. Psychoanal Rev 14:268–280, 1927

Chazan R: Group analytic therapy with schizophrenic outpatients. Group 17:164–178, 1993

Coons WH: Interaction and insight in group psychotherapy. Can J Psychol 11:1–8, 1957

Dobson DJG, McDougall G, Busheikin J, et al: Effects of social skills training and social milieu treatment on symptoms of schizophrenia. Psychiatric Services 46:376–380, 1995

Donlan PT, Rada RT, Knight SW: A therapeutic aftercare setting for "refractory" chronic schizophrenic patients. Am J Psychiatry 130:682–684, 1973

Douglas MS, Mueser KT: Teaching conflict resolution skills to the chronically ill. Behav Modif 14:519–547, 1990

Drake RE, Sederer LI: The adverse effects of intensive treatment of chronic schizophrenia. Compr Psychiatry 27:313–326, 1986

Engel GL: The clinical application of the biopsychosocial model. Am J Psychiatry 137:535–544, 1980

Erickson RC: Heterogeneous groups: a legitimate alternative. Group 10:21–26, 1986

Fenn HH, Dinaburg D: Didactic group psychotherapy with chronic schizophrenics. Int J Group Psychother 31:443–452, 1981

Frank JD: Group Therapy in the Mental Hospital. Washington, DC, American Psychiatric Association Mental Hospital Service, 1955

Geczy B, Sultenfuss J: Group psychotherapy on state hospital admissions wards. Int J Group Psychother 45:1–15, 1995

Gordon J, Adebakin D, Jones A: "The depot group": mutual injection of emotion in community psychiatry. Group Analysis 27:449–457, 1994

Gould E, Garrigues CS, Scheikowitz K: Interaction in hospitalized patient-led psychotherapy groups. Am J Psychother 29:383–390, 1975

Gruber LN: Group techniques for acutely psychotic inpatients. Group 2:31–39, 1978

Gunn RC: A use of videotape with inpatient therapy groups. Int J Group Psychother 28:365–370, 1978

Hegarty JD, Baldessarini RJ, Tohen M, et al: One hundred years of schizophrenia: a meta-analysis of the outcome literature. Am J Psychiatry 151:1409–1416, 1994

Hierholzer RW, Liberman RP: Successful living: a social skills and problem-solving group for the chronic mentally ill. Hosp Community Psychiatry 37:913–918, 1986

Horowitz MJ, Weisberg PS: Techniques for the group psychotherapy of acute psychosis. Int J Group Psychother 16:42–50, 1966

Johnson D, Geller J, Gordon J, et al: Group psychotherapy with schizophrenic patients: the pairing group. Int J Group Psychother 36:75–96, 1986

Josephs L, Juman L: The application of self psychology principles to long-term group therapy with schizophrenic inpatients. Group 9:21–30, 1985

Kahn EM: Group treatment interventions for schizophrenics. Int J Group Psychother 34:149–153, 1984

Kanas N: Group therapy with schizophrenics: a review of controlled studies. Int J Group Psychother 36:339–351, 1986a

Kanas N: Therapy groups with schizophrenics: response to Dr. Parloff. Int J Group Psychother 36:597–601, 1986b

Kanas N, Rogers M, Kreth E, et al: The effectiveness of group psychotherapy during the first three weeks of hospitalization: a controlled study. J Nerv Ment Dis 168:487–492, 1980

Kaplan HI, Sadock BJ: Comprehensive Textbook of Psychiatry, 5th Edition. Baltimore, MD, Williams & Wilkins, 1989

Kapur R: Measuring the effects of group interpretations with the severely mentally ill. Group Analysis 26:411–432, 1993

Kibel HD: A conceptual model for short-term inpatient group psychotherapy. Am J Psychiatry 138:74–80, 1981

Kibel HD: Inpatient group psychotherapy: where treatment philosophies converge, in The Yearbook of Psychoanalysis, Vol 2. Edited by Langs R. New York, Gardner Press, 1987, pp 94–116

Kibel HD: The therapeutic use of splitting: the role of the mother-group in therapeutic differentiation and practicing, in Psychoanalytic Group Theory and Therapy. Edited by Tuttman S. Madison, CT, International Universities Press, 1991, pp 113–132

Klapman JW: The case for didactic group psychotherapy. Diseases of the Nervous System 11:35–41, 1950

Klapman JW: Clinical practices of group psychotherapy with psychotics. Int J Group Psychother 1:22–30, 1951

Klein RH: Inpatient group psychotherapy: practical considerations and special problems. Int J Group Psychother 27:201–214, 1977

Lawton JJ: The expanding horizon of group psychotherapy in schizophrenic convalescence. Int J Group Psychother 1:218–224, 1951

Lazell EW: The group treatment of dementia praecox. Psychoanal Rev 8:168–179, 1921

Leopold HS: Selective group approaches with psychotic patients in hospital settings. Am J Psychother 30:95–102, 1976

MacDonald WS, Blochberger CW, Maynard HM: Group therapy: a comparison of patient-led and staff-led groups on an open hospital ward. Psychiatr Q 38 (suppl):290–303, 1964

Malawista KL, Malawista PL: Modified group-as-a-whole psychotherapy with chronic psychotic patients. Bull Menninger Clin 52:114–125, 1988

Marsh LC: An experiment in the group treatment of patients at the Worcester State Hospital. Ment Hygiene 17:397–416, 1933

Maxmen JS: An educative model for inpatient group therapy. Int J Group Psychother 28:321–338, 1978

McIntosh D, Stone WN, Grace M: The flexible boundaried group: format, techniques, and patients' perceptions. Int J Group Psychother 41:49–64, 1991

Milders CFA: Kernberg's object-relations theory and the group psychotherapy of psychosis. Group Analysis 27:419–432, 1994

Misunis MA, Feist BJ, Thorkelsson JG, et al: Outpatient groups for chronic psychiatric patients. Group 14:111–120, 1990

Pattison EM, Brissenden E, Wohl T: Assessing special effects of inpatient group psychotherapy. Int J Group Psychother 17:283–297, 1967

Pinney EL: Reactions of outpatient schizophrenics to group psychotherapy. Int J Group Psychother 6:147–151, 1956

Plante TG, Pinder SL, Howe D: Introducing the living with illness group: a specialized treatment for patients with chronic schizophrenic conditions. Group 12:198–204, 1988

Roback HB: Experimental comparison of outcome in insight- and noninsight-oriented therapy groups. J Consult Clin Psychol 38:411–417, 1972

Sandison R: Group therapy and drug therapy, in Group Psychotherapy and Group Function, Revised Edition. Edited by Rosenbaum M, Berger MM. New York, Basic Books, 1975, pp 608–621

Sandison R: The psychotic patient and psychotic conflict in group analysis. Group Analysis 24:73–83, 1991

Sandison R: Working with schizophrenics individually and in groups: understanding the psychotic process. Group Analysis 27:393–406, 1994

Schilder P: Results and problems of group psychotherapy in severe neuroses. Ment Hygiene 23:87–98, 1939

Semon RG, Goldstein N: The effectiveness of group psychotherapy with chronic schizophrenic patients and an evaluation of different therapeutic methods. Journal of Consulting Psychology 21:317–322, 1957

Semrad EV: Psychotherapy of the psychosis in a state hospital. Diseases of the Nervous System 9:105–111, 1948

Serok S, Rabin C, Spitz Y: Intensive Gestalt group therapy with schizophrenics. Int J Group Psychother 34:431–450, 1984

Slavson SR: Group psychotherapy and the nature of schizophrenia. Int J Group Psychother 11:3–32, 1961

Standish CT, Semrad EV: Group psychotherapy with psychotics. Journal of Psychiatric Social Work 20:143–150, 1951

Strassberg DS, Roback HB, Anchor KN, et al: Self-disclosure in group therapy with schizophrenics. Arch Gen Psychiatry 32:1259–1261, 1975

Takahashi T, Washington WP: A group-centered object relations approach to group psychotherapy with severely disturbed patients. Int J Group Psychother 41:79–96, 1991

Weiner MF: Outcome of psychoanalytically oriented group psychotherapy. Group 8:3–12, 1984

Wender L: The dynamics of group psychotherapy and its application. J Nerv Ment Dis 84:54–60, 1936

World Health Organization: The ICD-10 Classification of Mental and Behavioural Disorders. Geneva, Switzerland, World Health Organization, 1992

Yalom ID: Inpatient Group Psychotherapy. New York, Basic Books, 1983

Yehoshua R, Kellermann PF, Calev A, et al: Group psychotherapy with inpatient chronic schizophrenics. Isr J Psychiatry Relat Sci 22:185–190, 1985

CHAPTER 3

Theoretical Issues

*R*osegrant (1988) argued that there are three major theoretical approaches that can be used in conducting inpatient therapy groups with severely mentally ill patients: educative, psychodynamic, and interpersonal. In Chapter 2, I found that these same three orientations have historically characterized the use of groups with schizophrenic patients dating back to 1921. In this chapter, I describe the three approaches more fully, citing a contemporary example of each. This is followed by a discussion of the pros and cons of these theoretical orientations. After this, the integrative treatment model that is described in this book is introduced from a theoretical perspective; it is compared and contrasted with the three preceding orientations.

Educative Approach

The educative approach stems from the work of Lazell (1921) and Marsh (1933), and its basic clinical elements are shown in Table 3–1. This orientation focuses on the biological aspects of schizophrenia, viewing the patients as suffering from a major mental disease with constitutional and genetic components. This orientation holds that the main goals of group therapy with schizophrenic patients are to help them learn strategies of coping with the symptoms of their illness (e.g., hallucinations and delusions) and the everyday problems that are caused by the disease. This is done through lectures, advice from the therapist, question-and-answer periods, problem solving, group exercises such as role-playing, and homework assignments that are completed between the sessions. Although the discussions that follow the lectures allow the members to interact with one another, the content usually relates to the topic that was presented or to the patients' symptoms and their relief. Issues involving the unconscious, past conflicts, and transference interpretations rarely are considered. The time focus is the present, particularly as it relates to the manifestations and sequelae of the disease.

Contemporary proponents of the educative approach are Fenn and Dinaburg (1981). They stated their basic orientation as follows: "The availability of a proved pharmacologic treatment for schizophrenia and recent research into the disorder's biological basis puts the condition squarely in the category of a medical disease" (p. 450). They described two formats for treating schizophrenic outpatients in group therapy. The first utilizes four weekly sessions that last for 1 hour each: 30 minutes of a didactic presentation followed by 30 minutes of discussion. Arguing that a major cause of hospitalization is stopping antipsychotic medications, they stated that the goals of the group are "to maximize patient autonomy, increase patient knowledge of medications, build a support system, strengthen the therapeutic alliance, and thereby encourage compliance" (p. 445). Using a blackboard, the leader lectures on the following topics: 1) a biologically based definition of schizophrenia, 2) brain chemistry and the dopamine

Table 3–1.   Group therapy with schizophrenic patients: educative approach

Disease emphasis	The biological and phenomenological aspects of schizophrenia (e.g., hallucinations and delusions)
Group goals	To help patients learn to cope with the symptoms of their disease and the real problems that they cause
Examples of techniques	Lectures, advice giving, question-and-answer periods, problem solving, role-playing, homework
Time focus	Present

hypothesis, 3) the therapeutic effects and side effects of antipsychotic medications, and 4) characteristics of a relapse. This sequence is followed by monthly alumni sessions.

The second format is used for patients who are more stable, are taking their medications, and have been in the clinic for a longer period of time. It utilizes a biweekly group approach composed of hourly sessions that consist of a 30-minute lecture-discussion, followed by the serving of doughnuts, and then a discussion of each patient's medications. The leader jots down major points on a blackboard and usually chooses the topics for discussion, which generally focus on phenomenological aspects of schizophrenia and on medications. During the discussions, the leader tries to "engage the withdrawn patients and foster feelings of identification and common purpose" (p. 446).

In both of these formats, the therapists present themselves as experts who are trying to help the patients learn about their illness. Schizophrenia is considered from the framework of the medical model. The atmosphere is didactic, and the topics are practical and introduced in a seminar style. Groups utilizing these treatment formats have been followed for more than a year, and the authors concluded that they have made a positive impact on the patients.

Psychodynamic Approach

This orientation may be traced back to early psychoanalytic concepts as they were applied to groups of schizophrenic patients by Schilder (1939), Semrad and his colleagues (Semrad 1948; Standish and Semrad 1951), and staff at the Brooklyn State Hospital (Lawton 1951, Pinney 1956). The basic ideas of this approach are shown in Table 3–2. Although not ignoring the biological and social aspects of the disease, the focus is on early psychological conflicts, deficiencies, and arrests that result in maladaptive behaviors and ego function deficits. These vulnerabilities predispose schizophrenic patients to develop the characteristic signs and symptoms of the disease as a result of stress, maturational challenges, or the vicissitudes of life. The traditional goals of psychodynamic group therapy with these patients are to help them gain an understanding of how long-standing psychological problems and maladaptive behaviors interfere with their lives and to improve their ego functions through this understanding and the corrective emotional experience that results from participating in the group. Techniques that are used include open discussions whose topics are generated by the group members, the uncovering of important unconscious issues, and interpretations of transference reactions. The time focus is the past, because the therapist wants to help the patients understand the psychological antecedents of their disease to help them strengthen their ego functions and improve their lives in the present. The psychodynamic approach can be very intense, and the resulting anxiety can lead to regression and exacerbation of symptoms. For this reason, some psychodynamically oriented group therapists advocate the addition of supportive comments and directive techniques to help psychotic patients weather the storms of therapy.

The object relations model of Kernberg (1976) is an example of a current psychodynamic approach that has lent itself to group therapy. According to this model, patients who have developed psychotic character structures are unable to differentiate internal self and object representations clearly, which results in a blurring of ego boundaries. Consequently, a "bad" aggressively linked self-object unit, which is relatively undifferentiated, is split off, denied, and extruded from a "good" pleasurable self-object constellation. The latter helps the patients relate to their environment in a primitive but organized manner.

Table 3–2.   Group therapy with schizophrenic patients: psychodynamic approach

Disease emphasis	The psychological aspects of schizophrenia
Group goals	To help patients gain an understanding of how long-standing psychological problems and maladaptive behaviors interfere with their lives, with the aim of lessening their impact and improving ego functions
Examples of techniques	Open discussion, exploration of the unconscious, transference interpretations
Time focus	Past

Kibel (1981, 1987, 1991) applied this theory to group therapy. He stated that

> Decompensation into acute psychosis can be viewed as a regressive refusion of the "good" self and object constellation with concomitant intrusion of the aggressively linked, self-object unit into this libidinal core. Such disintegration of overall psychic structures produces fragmentation of the experience of oneself; pathological fusion of fragments of self and object representations produces new units that are fantastic in nature. The latter account for much of the symptomatology as these are projected onto the external world. (Kibel 1981, p. 77)

As a result, self-reflective capacity and reality testing are impaired.

In this psychodynamic approach, small groups of not more than four members are recommended for severely regressed and psychotic patients. Patients who are less acutely ill can be treated in larger groups of six to eight members. In either case, the environment should be safe and supportive.

Kibel (1991) believes that in the therapy group, primitive patterns of relatedness, such as the search for a need-gratifying maternal image, are activated. The resulting "mother-group" creates a nurturing environment that helps the members identify with the group and tolerate their own aggressive introjects so that splitting can occur in a planned, organized manner. This allows the patients to reprocess and internalize their projected fantasies. Thus, the more supportive and cohesive the group environment, the more secure the patients will be in exposing these "bad" aspects of themselves.

> The danger in this approach is that cohesion and the attachment to the group entity become overly sustaining for these patients and, thereby, makes eventual separation from treatment difficult. However, this may be a small price to pay for patients with such severe impairment of functioning. They may be "lifers" in treatment in any event. (p. 121)

To create this group environment, the therapist needs to be active and directive in helping the patients interact and support one another.

Like a symphonic conductor, the therapist must orchestrate the flow of the group. He must take the initiative to encourage discussion and even occasionally introduce topics. He must bring in relevant material from previous sessions and pick up on the subtler aspects of their conversation and behavior. (Kibel 1991, p. 122)

At times, comments are made to the group as a whole to promote cohesion and mutuality. Unlike some other psychoanalytically oriented group approaches, Kibel's method does not place a strong emphasis on insight. Instead, through the actions of the therapist, the patients are encouraged to confront each other's distortions, improve their interactions, and reprocess and internalize their projected fantasies.

Interpersonal Approach

This orientation stems from the work of Frank and his colleagues (Frank 1955; Powdermaker and Frank 1953). The basic features of the model are given in Table 3–3. Although not disputing the presence of biological and psychological factors, the main emphasis is on the interpersonal aspects of schizophrenia. The patients are viewed as being socially isolated and as reacting maladaptively with others. Consequently, the goals of the group are to help the members become less isolated and to improve their ability to relate. This is accomplished through discussions of current inter-

Table 3–3.   Group therapy with schizophrenic patients: interpersonal approach

Disease emphasis	The interpersonal aspects of schizophrenia
Group goals	To help patients become less socially isolated and to improve their ability to relate appropriately with others
Examples of techniques	Discussions of interpersonal problems, encouraging patient interactions in the group (e.g., structured exercises, maintaining eye contact), here-and-now interpretations of member interactions
Time focus	Present

personal problems and ways to deal with them. In addition, the therapist pays close attention to any inappropriate interactions that take place during the sessions. By pointing these out as they occur in the so-called here and now, other patients can comment along with the therapist, and the impact is immediate and powerful. Thus, the time focus is the present, and change occurs as a result of interpersonal feedback that is given in the here and now of the group. Not only do schizophrenic patients learn ways of relating better with others, but they also are forced to challenge some of the delusional material behind their general feelings of mistrust, their suspicions of others, and their rationalization of being isolated. Because much of what is curative in the interpersonal approach depends on group member interactions, these are encouraged through a variety of techniques, such as using structured interpersonal exercises and asking patients to look at each other when they are talking.

A current advocate of the interpersonal approach is Yalom (1975, 1983). He views schizophrenic patients as doing better in groups that are supportive and undemanding and provide an opportunity for a successful experience. He believes that a reality-focused, structured approach is better than one that is insight oriented and unstructured. Anxiety should be kept to a minimum. The therapists should be active, open, and encouraging. They must help patients develop social skills that will allow them to become engaged with others outside of the group, and they should focus on here-and-now interactions whenever possible.

As an example, he described a "lower-level" group format for regressed psychotic patients on short-term inpatient units (Yalom 1983). The group is open and consists of four to seven members. It meets five times a week for 45-minute sessions. The sessions are highly organized, with a basic plan that consists of an orientation (2–5 minutes), a warm-up (5–10 minutes), structured exercises (20–30 minutes), and a review of the session (5–10 minutes). The orientation serves to initiate new members and to clarify issues for continuing members who may be psychotic or confused. "The warm-up consists of one or more brief structured exercises which provide a gentle beginning to the group. It decreases anticipatory anxiety and permits each member to engage in brief, light, and nonthreatening interaction" (p. 287). Examples of warm-up exercises include throwing a balloon around the group room, making comments about a fellow member's appearance, or saying something personal about oneself.

The bulk of the session consists of two or three short (5–15 minute) structured exercises. Most of these require some self-disclosure and member interaction. Yalom (1983) stated that "the most effective type of exercise, in my experience, has been a pairing exercise which combines solo activity, dyadic interaction, and total group interaction" (pp. 290–291). For example, members may be given sheets of paper with statements to complete that describe important characteristics of themselves. These sometimes relate to an important group theme for that session (e.g., separation, anger, isolation). When this has been accomplished, the patients are asked to trade papers with a "buddy." Each member of the pair then asks for clarification or elaboration of what the other has written. The group re-forms, and each person reads aloud what his or her partner wrote, along with what has been learned in the clarification period. Other types of exercise include asking patients to make empathic comments about one another or to give each other feedback on ways to change an undesirable trait. Playing an interpersonal game also can be helpful. "Games may relieve tension, provide a light respite between more challenging tasks, increase member interaction, improve social skills, and augment group cohesiveness" (pp. 301–302). Note that all of these exercises encourage the patients to interact with each other in real time, either in dyads or in the larger group, even though the issue being discussed may not be interpersonal in nature. Thus, they are breaking out of their shell of isolation and practicing important social skills that can be transferred to the outside.

During the review, the therapist asks the members first to reconstruct what happened during the session, then to evaluate it. They also evaluate each other in terms of who was most active, who took risks, who was most supportive, and so on. This review has many advantages, such as alleviating confusion, encouraging the patients to assume responsibility for their treatment, and increasing their attention span. In addition, it asks the members to examine their interactions in a self-reflecting loop that encourages them to relate in the here and now.

> Since they know that they will be asked to review the meeting in a comprehensive manner, they make an attempt to attend as

fully as possible to their own participation and to that of the other members. The more that patients learn to live in the present, rather than in the future or the past, the more satisfaction will they derive from life, and the more successful will they be in engaging other individuals. (Yalom 1983, p. 307)

Theoretical Analysis

Theoretically speaking, each of the three models mentioned has strengths and weaknesses when it comes to dealing with psychotic schizophrenic patients in therapy groups. The educative approach helps the patients learn strategies of coping with the symptoms of their disease. They gain cognitive information that gives them a sense of control and mastery over their disorder. The sessions are structured and the agenda is clear. The techniques are largely didactic (e.g., lectures, advice giving, question-and-answer periods, problem solving, role-playing, homework). This results in a safe, supportive, and familiar classroomlike environment. The topics are relevant to their needs as schizophrenic individuals. Discussions usually are related to the topics, and they give the patients an opportunity to clarify points that were made, to express their feelings, and to interact minimally with one another.

However, the educative approach does not pay adequate attention to the psychosocial needs of these patients. The basic assumption is that schizophrenia is a biological disease, and this is where the emphasis is placed. Typically, for example, more is said about reducing symptoms through the use of medications than through the use of psychosocial strategies, even though the latter have been found to be useful in helping patients cope with psychotic experiences (Breier and Strauss 1983; Cohen and Berk 1985; Corrigan and Storzbach 1993; Dobson et al. 1995; Falloon and Talbot 1981; Kanas and Barr 1984). Although the presence of a lecture sequence and the inherent structure of the sessions help minimize anxiety, they do not provide enough flexibility to deal with the needs of new patients or with the sudden crises that affect continuing patients. For example, a new patient may arrive in the group having problems with auditory hallucinations, but he or she would have to wait until this issue is scheduled before being able to discuss it at any length. Similarly, it would be possible for a patient to attend such a group and not have the opportunity to express his or her despair about having a chronic mental illness. In addition, techniques that encourage patients to interact with one another are not emphasized, which is a major problem for people who are isolative and have deficits in social skills.

The psychodynamic approach pays special attention to the psychological needs of the patients. The discussions are open in that they allow the members to introduce the topics that will be addressed during the session. This allows a number of issues to be considered, and it provides a forum for any acute problem that affects a member to be discussed at the next available session. By uncovering past conflicts and maladaptive behaviors that have affected them throughout their lives, the patients can begin to see how these have contributed to their current problems. Together with the corrective emotional experience that results from participating in the group, this knowledge strengthens ego functions and allows the members to behave more appropriately.

However, the psychodynamic approach is quite intensive. By its very nature, it can lead to the uncovering of unpleasant memories and affects that produce anxiety, regression, and exacerbation of symptoms in psychotic patients (Drake and Sederer 1986; Geczy and Sultenfuss 1995; Kanas et al. 1980; MacDonald et al. 1964; Pattison et al. 1967; Strassberg et al. 1975; Weiner 1984). Sensitive, dynamically oriented clinicians (Kibel 1981, 1987, 1991; Takahashi and Washington 1991) have recognized this and have attempted to restrict the amount of uncovering that is done and to add support and direction to their approach. However, most psychodynamic groups lack structure and pull for the kinds of issues that are more properly addressed in nonpsychotic populations. In addition, transference-oriented interpretations have been associated with low patient responsiveness ratings in groups of severely mentally ill patients (Kapur 1993). Finally, not enough attention is paid to the importance of member interactions and to the here and now in these groups. Schizophrenic patients have major problems with relationships, and an opportunity is lost if the group process is not utilized to address these problems in real time.

The interpersonal approach focuses on the isolation and relationship problems that are experienced by schizophrenic patients. Discussions address these issues and consider ways of dealing with them. Because the emphasis is on current problems, what is learned in the group has immediate relevance to interpersonal issues outside of the group. Techniques are employed that encourage the members to interact with one another. Thus, they are able to practice improving their social skills using the group as a laboratory. Maladaptive interactions can be observed and commented on in the here and now of the sessions, and this immediacy is a powerful change factor. The interpersonal approach also creates an environment that emphasizes socially appropriate contacts between the group members.

However, learning to cope with psychotic symptoms, strengthening certain ego functions, such as reality testing ability and impulse control, and discussing nonrelational psychological problems are minimized in this approach, even though these are important issues that should be addressed in the group. In addition, whereas reliance on structured exercises may be useful for some extremely regressed inpatients, they are not necessary for all schizophrenic patients, even in hospital settings (Geczy and Sultenfuss 1995). Psychotic individuals may have fragile egos, but discussions can be directed in such a way so as to allow freedom of expression without compromising patient safety, as is seen in Chapter 5. Unnecessary structure infantilizes patients and prevents important issues from being raised. Finally, although a here-and-now focus is extremely valuable, it can be intensive. Like too much uncovering, it can make patients anxious, particularly in situations where it leads to the expression of anger between group members. In such a case, it may be necessary to direct the group's attention to the past or to outside relationships to defuse the situation.

Integrative Approach

The approach advocated in this book takes a biopsychosocial perspective of schizophrenia and is an integration of the previous three theoretical orientations. Although this model is described more fully in the next three chapters, it is useful here to compare it theoretically with the educative, psychodynamic, and interpersonal approaches. This is done in Table 3–4.

Like the educative approach, a major goal of the integrative model is to help the patients learn ways of coping with the symptoms of schizophrenia. Patients are able to learn about medications from their doctors, but they usually do not have much of an opportunity to learn about important psychosocial strategies that may help them deal with the phenomenology of their disease. Consequently, although these groups occasionally discuss medications, a more important focus is the sharing of various psychosocial coping strategies between patients during the discussions. Also like the educative approach, the discussion topics are focused on the needs of schizophrenic patients, and care is given to avoid extraneous issues. Finally, there is an emphasis on making the group a safe place for the patients through the use of struc-

Table 3–4.   Group therapy with schizophrenic patients: similarities of integrative approach with other approaches

---

• **Educative approach**

Major goal is to learn ways of coping with psychotic symptoms (but psychosocial strategies are given more emphasis than medication strategies).

Discussion topics focus on the needs of schizophrenic patients.

Therapists create a safe environment through the group structure (which in our groups is incorporated into the discussions by the therapists' interventions).

• **Psychodynamic approach**

Groups are discussion oriented and discussions are open (i.e., patients generate the topics and there are no lectures or formal structured exercises).

Long-term maladaptive problems may be examined in reference to current problems.

Ego functions are strengthened.

• **Interpersonal approach**

Major goal is to become less isolated and improve relationships with others.

Members are encouraged to interact with each other during the sessions.

Maladaptive interactions are examined in the here and now of the group.

---

ture. However, this is not built into the sessions in terms of time demands (i.e., so much time for lectures, so much time for discussion, and so on); instead, the therapists provide structure through their interventions in the discussions. Safety is uppermost in the leader's mind, and a well-placed comment can reinforce a productive issue or block the course of an issue that may become explosive or anxiety producing.

Like the psychodynamic approach, the integrative model is discussion oriented, and the discussions are open. This means that the patients are able to generate the topics from session to session, as long as the topic area is congruent with the goals of the group. This provides flexibility and allows important issues to come up without fear that they will upset an agenda. Lectures and formal structured exercises are not a major feature in the groups, because it is believed that patients can learn a great deal from one another in open discussions if the therapist creates an environment that is goal directed and encourages the patients to interact with one another. Also like the psychodynamic model, the integrative approach sometimes examines the ways that long-standing maladaptive behaviors are related to present-day problems. However, the focus generally is more on the present than on the past, and this longitudinal look occurs more in the long-term outpatient groups than in the short-term outpatient or in-patient groups. Finally, the techniques are oriented toward strengthening ego functions that are particularly fragile in schizophrenic patients, such as reality testing and reality sense. Uncovering techniques (e.g., exploring the unconscious, interpreting transference) are avoided because these raise anxiety and are too intensive for most schizophrenic patients.

Like the interpersonal approach, a major goal of the integrative model is to help patients become less isolated and improve their relationships with others. This is done in part through the group discussions, which frequently deal with interpersonal themes. In addition, the patients are encouraged to interact with one another using a variety of techniques, which are elaborated on in Chapter 5. Thus, they practice important social skills that can be utilized outside of the group. Another similarity with the interpersonal approach is the use of the here and now to point out maladaptive interactions that are observed between members in the group. When done supportively, this can show patients how they get into trouble with others, and it can lead to discussions of ways to improve their interactions. It should be stressed that the theoretical considerations of the integrative approach considered here are the end result of research work dating back to 1975. We did not begin with a fully developed theory or set of clinical techniques. Rather, we started with a basic clinical strategy that focused on enhancing coping skills and improving relationships, then tested it empirically through research activities. What was learned was then fed back into clinical activities, and new researchable ideas resulted. These in turn were studied, and the findings again were incorporated into practice. Thus, over time, a treatment model evolved from the research, which began to take on the characteristics of other clinical approaches. This empirical work is described in Chapter 7. In the next chapter, I discuss the important clinical features that characterize the integrative model.

References

Breier A, Strauss JS: Self-control in psychotic disorders. Arch Gen Psychiatry 40:1141–1145, 1983

Cohen CI, Berk LA: Personal coping styles of schizophrenic outpatients. Hosp Community Psychiatry 36:407–410, 1985

Corrigan PW, Storzbach DM: Behavioral interventions for alleviating psychotic symptoms. Hosp Community Psychiatry 44:341–347, 1993

Dobson DJG, McDougall G, Busheikin J, et al: Effects of social skills training and social milieu treatment on symptoms of schizophrenia. Psychiatric Services 46:376–380, 1995

Drake RE, Sederer LI: The adverse effects of intensive treatment of chronic schizophrenia. Compr Psychiatry 27:313–326, 1986

Falloon IRH, Talbot RE: Persistent auditory hallucinations: coping mechanisms and implications for management. Psychol Med 11:329–339, 1981

Fenn HH, Dinaburg D: Didactic group psychotherapy with chronic schizophrenics. Int J Group Psychother 31:443–452, 1981

Frank JD: Group Therapy in the Mental Hospital. Washington, DC, American Psychiatric Association Mental Hospital Service, 1955

Geczy B, Sultenfuss J: Group psychotherapy on state hospital admission wards. Int J Group Psychother 45:1–15, 1995

Kanas N, Barr MA: Self-control of psychotic productions in schizophrenics. Arch Gen Psychiatry 41:919–920, 1984

Kanas N, Rogers M, Kreth E, et al: The effectiveness of group psychotherapy during the first three weeks of hospitalization: a controlled study. J Nerv Ment Dis 168:487–492, 1980

Kapur R: Measuring the effects of group interpretations with the severely mentally ill. Group Analysis 26:411–432, 1993

Kernberg OF: Object-Relations Theory and Clinical Psychoanalysis. New York, Jason Aronson, 1976

Kibel HD: A conceptual model for short-term inpatient group psychotherapy. Am J Psychiatry 138:74–80, 1981

Kibel HD: Inpatient group psychotherapy: where treatment philosophies converge, in The Yearbook of Psychoanalysis, Vol 2. Edited by Langs R. New York, Gardner Press, 1987, pp 94–116

Kibel HD: The therapeutic use of splitting: the role of the mother-group in therapeutic differentiation and practicing, in Psychoanalytic Group Theory and Therapy. Edited by Tuttman S. Madison, CT, International Universities Press, 1991, pp 113–132

Lawton JJ: The expanding horizon of group psychotherapy in schizophrenic convalescence. Int J Group Psychother 1:218–224, 1951

Lazell EW: The group treatment of dementia praecox. Psychoanal Rev 8:168–179, 1921

MacDonald WS, Blochberger CW, Maynard HM: Group therapy: a comparison of patient-led and staff-led groups on an open hospital ward. Psychiatr Q 38 (suppl):290–303, 1964

Marsh LC: An experiment in the group treatment of patients at the Worcester State Hospital. Ment Hygiene 17:397–416, 1933

Pattison EM, Brissenden E, Wohl T: Assessing special effects of inpatient group psychotherapy. Int J Group Psychother 17:283–297, 1967

Pinney EL: Reactions of outpatient schizophrenics to group psychotherapy. Int J Group Psychother 6:147–151, 1956

Powdermaker FB, Frank JD: Group Psychotherapy: Studies in Methodology of Research and Therapy. Cambridge, MA, Harvard University Press, 1953

Rosegrant J: A dynamic/expressive approach to brief inpatient group psychotherapy. Group 12:103–112, 1988

Schilder P: Results and problems of group psychotherapy in severe neuroses. Ment Hygiene 23:87–98, 1939

Semrad EV: Psychotherapy of the psychosis in a state hospital. Diseases of the Nervous System 9:105–111, 1948

Standish CT, Semrad EV: Group psychotherapy with psychotics. Journal of Psychiatric Social Work 20:143–150, 1951

Strassberg DS, Roback HB, Anchor KN, et al: Self-disclosure in group therapy with schizophrenics. Arch Gen Psychiatry 32:1259–1261, 1975

Takahashi T, Washington WP: A group-centered object relations approach to group psychotherapy with severely disturbed patients. Int J Group Psychother 41:79–96, 1991

Weiner MF: Outcome of psychoanalytically oriented group psychotherapy. Group 8:3–12, 1984

Yalom ID: The Theory and Practice of Group Psychotherapy, 2nd Edition. New York, Basic Books, 1975

Yalom ID: Inpatient Group Psychotherapy. New York, Basic Books, 1983

CHAPTER 4

Clinical Issues: Group Format

*I*n setting up any therapy group, a number of questions need to be answered. Who will participate, and what are their major problems? What are the goals of the group? How many therapists need to be involved to accomplish these goals? How often will the group meet, and for how long? What is the optimal number of patients? Should medications be given concomitantly? These issues of group format must be resolved before the first patient is screened. In this chapter, I consider these issues in terms of the integrative group model, providing the structure for the clinical strategies that are described in the next chapter.

Treatment Goals

As mentioned earlier, schizophrenic patients suffer from a number of severe symptoms throughout much of their adult lives. Auditory hallucinations, persecutory and referential delusions, thought insertion and thought broadcasting, loose associations, catatonic behavior, negative symptoms—these and many other experiences interfere with the ability of schizophrenic patients to function in the real world and are a source of distress and dysphoria. In addition, these patients experience a number of problems interacting with other people. Sometimes this is due to the interference of psychotic symptoms. Many schizophrenic patients have never learned basic interpersonal skills, however, and they display a fear and distrust of others or a naïveté that allows others to abuse them. As a result, these patients become guarded and isolative, and this further compounds their difficulties. For these reasons, the integrative approach for treating schizophrenic patients in therapy groups focuses on two major treatment goals. The first aims to help the members cope with their symptoms. For most patients, this means learning to test reality and deal with psychotic symptoms. Although antipsychotic medications are useful in helping patients deal with these experiences, a number of authors have reported that psychosocial interventions also are helpful (Breier and Strauss 1983; Cohen and Berk 1985; Corrigan and Storzbach 1993; Dobson et al. 1995; Falloon and Talbot 1981; Kanas and Barr 1984). In our schizophrenic groups, I have found that when psychotic symptoms are perceived to be unpleasant and foreign (i.e., ego-alien), the patients are motivated to discuss coping strategies that will minimize their influence. When they are perceived to be acceptable and natural (i.e., ego-syntonic), the patients first need to understand that most people do not have these experiences and that the symptoms are part of an illness. When psychotic symptoms are perceived to be comforting and useful (e.g., helpful advice from auditory hallucinations), this creates a motivational problem because the patients may be loath to give them up. In this case, the focus of treatment should be on helping the patients understand how the experiences are interfering with their lives, such as giving them unrealistic advice or driving people away from them.

The second major goal of treatment is to help the group members learn ways to improve their interpersonal relationships. This can range from simply making contact with people in casual situations to taking appropriate risks in trusting others to form longstanding friendships. As an interactional form of treatment, group therapy is particularly useful in improving interpersonal relationships in two ways. First, patients can discuss their isolation and the problems they have in relating with others and consider solutions to correct these problems. Second, in the process of discussing these issues during each session, the patients are practicing and improving their interpersonal skills in a controlled environment that is regulated by the therapist. Healthy interactions are reinforced, and these can be generalized to the patients' interpersonal lives outside of the group setting.

The relative importance of the two group goals and the frequency with which they are considered depend on the setting and history of the group. This is shown in Table 4–1. On acute-care inpatient units, where the schizophrenic patients are psychotic and where the groups are open (i.e., new members are added as they are admitted to the ward), learning ways of testing reality and coping with psychotic experiences are important and timely. Continuing members, especially those who are close to being discharged, can give encouragement and advice to new members about ways to deal with these issues. Relationship problems usually are discussed from the perspective of being caused by acute psychotic symptoms, and the focus is more on how interpersonal problems affect the members in the group and on the ward than on how they affect the patients outside of the hospital.

In newly formed or short-term outpatient groups that have a relatively consistent membership once they begin (so-called closed or slow-open groups), the patients are less psychotic than in the acute-care hospital setting. Consequently, there is more of

Table 4–1.   Effects of setting and history on the two major group goals

Setting and history	Effects on group goals
Open groups on acute-care inpatient units	The main focus is on helping the members test reality and cope with psychotic symptoms.
	Current interpersonal problems are discussed from the perspective of being sequelae of psychotic symptoms.
Closed newly formed or short-term outpatient groups	Coping with symptoms of schizophrenia and improving interpersonal relationships are discussed equally with reference to life both inside and outside the group.
Closed long-standing groups, inpatient or outpatient	Coping with symptoms of schizophrenia is discussed less often than improving interpersonal relationships.
	Long-standing problems and maladaptive patterns of relating with others are discussed with reference to their impact on current functioning.

a balance between issues related to schizophrenic symptoms and to poor interpersonal relationships. In addition, the patient's life outside of the clinical setting is discussed, although once again the focus is on practical problems that are current and immediate. For example, the distractions of auditory hallucinations or difficulties relating with a spouse are considered as they influence the members at the present time in their lives.

In closed groups that have met for several months, where the members have become cohesive and where they have dealt with immediate psychotic and interpersonal issues, it becomes more relevant to look at long-standing problems. Although ways to cope with symptom quality and intensity may be discussed, more group time is spent focusing on long-term maladaptive patterns of relating with others. In addition, patients have learned to trust each other, and issues that raise anxiety are better dealt with. Although the patients' past lives outside of the group (the there and then) may be considered, the issues that are raised are brought into the present and related to what may be affecting the members in the group (the here and now) or in their current life outside of the group. The idea is to help the patients through the corrective emotional experience that results from the group environment and through a generalization of this experience to the outside. Hopefully, this will correct long-standing deficits in ego functions and object relations, and the patients will feel more of a sense of mastery and control over their lives.

Patient Selection

Homogeneity of Patients

The cohesiveness of a group is affected by how homogeneous, or how similar, the members are to one another. However, the degree of similarity is relative, because homogeneity is a concept that can be expressed on a continuum in terms of many different parameters. For example, Erickson (1986) classified patients in terms of cognitive characteristics, Leopold (1976) constructed groups in terms of the members' ability to relate interpersonally, and Misunis et al. (1990) used general functional level based on a number of psychosocial factors. Using criteria such as these, similarities among patients are determined by psychological tests or by clinical judgment.

I have found diagnosis to be a useful construct in setting up schizophrenic groups, using standard criteria systems such as the *Diagnostic and Statistical Manual of Mental Disorders* (DSM-IV) (American Psychiatric Association 1994) and the *ICD-10 Classification of Mental and Behavioural Disorders* (World Health Organization 1992). At least in principle, a patient is included or excluded on the basis of meeting a set of clinical criteria that are objective and well known to mental health professionals and students. This results in a fair degree of homogeneity, because most of the group members have schizophrenia or a related condition.

In short-term inpatient groups composed of acutely psychotic patients or in brief time-limited outpatient groups, this homogeneous focus offers several advantages. First, because patients have much in common, they are able to relate quickly to one another. This rapid development of cohesiveness is useful in settings where the patients can attend only a limited number of sessions (MacKenzie 1990, 1994). Second, specific clinical techniques can be employed that are particularly useful for these patients. For example, an approach that focuses on coping strategies for psychotic symptoms would be quite relevant, whereas it might be inappropriate and boring for group members who had never experienced a psychotic break. Finally, techniques can be avoided that might be harmful for the patients. For example, clinical strategies that try to stimulate the emergence of unconscious material (e.g., long silences, emphasis on past conflicts) may be useful for neurotic patients, but they may produce anxiety and regression in schizophrenic patients, which may increase psychotic symptoms (Drake and Sederer 1986; Geczy and Sultenfuss 1995; Kanas et al. 1980; MacDonald et al. 1964; Pattison et al. 1967; Strassberg et al. 1975; Weiner 1984).

Despite the clinical advantages, there may be a practical problem in establishing a homogeneous schizophrenic group in some inpatient and outpatient settings: not having enough patients who have this or a related diagnosis. Thus, one must consider forming a group with patients from two (or possibly more) different wards or clinics, which is workable provided that the staff from these different settings communicate with one another and ensure that all of the patients show up. It also helps if they communicate special problems to the therapist or, in groups using a co-therapy approach, if each of the leaders is from one of the units. Where homogeneous groups are not possible, heterogeneous mixtures of schizophrenic and nonschizophrenic patients may be tried. In inpatient settings, such groups sometimes consist of the patients and therapists from the same treatment team (Yalom 1983). In outpatient settings, the heterogeneous approach works best when all of the patients are clinically stable and are able to tolerate some degree of anxiety and regression. This usually results in a format that is supportive and focuses on current problems. The nonschizophrenic patients generally suffer from severe personality disorders or other chronic conditions, and they are fairly low functioning. These patients sometimes are very helpful to schizophrenic patients by providing reality-based advice and relatively undistorted feedback concerning hallucinations, delusions, and maladaptive relationships (de Bosset 1991). Such groups generally are found in clinics dealing with chronically mentally ill persons or in day treatment settings.

Inclusion and Exclusion Criteria

Table 4–2 shows various inclusion and exclusion criteria in terms of diagnosis. In terms of DSM-IV criteria, ideal group patients would be suffering from any of the subtypes of schizophrenia or schizophreniform, schizoaffective, or delusional disorders. In chronic care settings, nonpsychotic severely mentally ill patients may be included in groups with clinically stable schizophrenic patients. Patients who have experienced psychotic episodes but

Table 4–2.   Group therapy inclusion and exclusion criteria in terms of diagnosis

Inclusion	Exclusion
Schizophrenic patients	High-functioning patients who have had psychotic episodes (e.g., bipolar, borderline, drug related)
Patients with schizophreniform, schizoaffective, or delusional disorders	
	Neurotic patients
Other chronically mentally ill patients (in groups with stable schizophrenic patients)	Patients with memory deficits
	Disruptive patients (e.g., antisocial personality)

who generally are high functioning do not benefit much from groups designed to meet the needs of schizophrenic patients. These include bipolar and borderline patients, those who have had an alcohol- or drug-related psychosis, and those who have experienced a brief psychotic disorder. Also contraindicated would be patients who require an insight-oriented, uncovering approach (e.g., neurotic patients), patients who have memory problems (e.g., those with severe organic brain syndrome), and those who would severely disrupt the therapeutic environment of any group (e.g., acute manic patients or patients with severe antisocial personality disorder).

In therapy groups composed largely of schizophrenic patients, each participant should be able to tolerate being in the treatment room for the entire session. Patients who are actively psychotic may be included as long as they are directable and are not too disruptive to the group process. In most cases, the group adjusts to minor disturbances, and the disruptive patient gains a sense of acceptance and comfort from the other group members. For example,

In one outpatient group, Albert would laugh inappropriately several times during each session. Frequently, he would try to suppress the laughter, but it would erupt explosively despite his best efforts. During an early session, Bob said that he felt Albert was laughing at him. Albert denied this, and I asked him why he kept laughing. He said that whenever he had a troubling thought or whenever people spoke about a topic that distressed him, he would deal with his feelings by thinking about a topic that was funny, and the resultant laughter made him feel better. I commented that this must be a handicap for him socially because people might misunderstand why he was laughing and believe, like Bob, that he was laughing at them. He agreed that it was a real problem, especially on buses when his sudden outbursts would draw attention and embarrass him. He then turned to Bob and tried to assure him that his laughter was nothing personal and that he could not control it. I asked the other patients what they thought of this. Bob said that he felt relief knowing why Albert was laughing. Carla said that she saw this as a real handicap for Albert but that she could live with it in the group now that she understood what was going on. From then on, Albert's laughter became part of the group climate and resulted in minimal disruption to the discussion.

Despite the diagnostic homogeneity of the groups, patients still vary in terms of degree of psychosis and type of symptoms. Whereas most patients have a preponderance of positive symptoms, such as hallucinations and delusions, some have negative symptoms, such as social withdrawal and lack of initiative. Although the former tend to be more verbally involved in the group, the latter also can benefit and should not be excluded.

For example,

> David, a quiet, withdrawn patient with several negative symptoms, was admitted to an inpatient group. Despite my attempts to involve him in the discussion, his comments were minimal, sometimes consisting of a yes or no, and sometimes just the statement: "I don't want to talk." Occasionally, David would say nothing, just respond with a blank stare. He particularly was loath to discuss anything dealing with emotions or psychotic symptoms. Despite this reluctance to talk, he was always alert and awake. During his last session before being discharged from the ward, we said goodbye to David, and I asked him if he had gotten anything out of the group. To my surprise, he said yes and proceeded to describe a couple of specific issues we had discussed previously that were meaningful to him. It was clear that he was listening, processing what was being said, and applying it to himself, even though he was not actively participating in the group discussions.

Demographic Issues

Our schizophrenic groups have included both men and women, people of all races and backgrounds, and both young and old patients. In this section, I consider these demographic factors as they apply to patient selection in groups conducted in general psychiatric settings. Issues that relate to specific culture-bound factors in the United States and abroad are discussed in Chapter 6.

Settings for our groups have included inpatient, outpatient, and day treatment programs at a veteran's hospital; medical school hospitals and clinics; public sector general hospitals in large cities; and a community mental health center. Groups have ranged from short-term (e.g., closed, outpatient, time-limited lasting up to 12 sessions) to long-term (e.g., open, inpatient, lasting for more than 15 years). In all of these settings with all of the groups mentioned, it was possible to train therapists to use the model presented in this book with great reliability and success. In fact, one study that examined an open inpatient group at two different points in time and compared it with a closed outpatient group found that the characteristics of the three group environments were the same, even though the patients, therapists, and process raters were different (Kanas and Smith 1990). Thus, the treatment approach has shown great robustness.

Because the model was developed for use with schizophrenic patients, and because the manifestations of this disorder are serious and protean, the demographic composition of the group is less important in determining the treatment approach than is the case with groups composed of other patients. This especially is true in acute-care settings, where the patients are quite disturbed and where coping with psychotic experiences is a key focus for the sessions. In addition, most of the patients in our groups are in the lower socioeconomic classes and have poor support systems, which is a common situation for schizophrenic patients (Africa and Schwartz 1992; Kaplan and Sadock 1989). However, this is not to say that differing patient demographics can be completely ignored as a factor in treatment. For example, in one inpatient study, it was found that significantly more patients below the median age of 29.5 years rated the group as being very helpful than those above the median age, and that significantly more nonparanoid schizophrenic patients found the group to be very helpful than those in the paranoid subtype (Kanas and Barr 1982). It is unclear what accounted for these effects of age and diagnostic subtype on the perceived helpfulness of the group in this study, but it suggests that the demographic characteristics of a group may influence its perceived helpfulness and possibly affect treatment outcome.

It is desirable to include both men and women in groups of schizophrenic patients. This is particularly important in outpatient settings, where the members are relatively stable and where issues involving feelings and relationships may be discussed with a fair degree of sophistication. In addition, having both men and women in the group allows for more relevant discussions involving issues related to gender and sex, and it creates a more characteristic microcosm of society. But even in inpatient settings, mixed-gender groups may be advantageous. For example, in Chapter 7, I present some pilot data that suggest that inpatient groups composed of both male and female schizophrenic patients may be more cohesive and less avoidant and tense than all-male groups. Although this explanation of the data is preliminary and confounded by other factors, it is consistent with the conclusions of others who advocate the advantages of mixed-gender therapy groups (Lazerson and Zilbach 1993; Taylor and Strassberg 1986).

As in any other therapy group, it makes good clinical sense to have at least two members of any demographic type in a group for schizophrenic patients. As MacKenzie (1990) said: "Every potential isolate needs to have someone with whom to identify" (p. 101); he calls this the Noah's Ark Principle. One black or Asian in a group of white people, or one woman in a group of men, sets up a situation where this individual can be scapegoated, isolated, or treated as special. This situation also may inhibit the participation of this person if he or she feels different from the others. Finally, it may perpetuate minority stereotyping. Dealing with these issues takes time and diverts the group away from its primary treatment goals.

Co-Therapy

Although a recent review of groups involving schizophrenic patients found that most had only one therapist (Kanas 1993), I believe that a co-therapy model using two therapists is better, for several reasons. First, groups of psychotic patients can be chaotic at times, with some members talking, others hallucinating, and still others gesturing or moving around the room. This is particularly true of groups located on acute-care hospital units. It sometimes is difficult for a therapist to get control of the group if he or she is trying to lead the discussion while also trying to attend to all of these distractions. With two leaders, one can focus on the topic at hand while the other monitors the behavior of the patients and takes any necessary actions. This is especially useful in potentially dangerous situations.

For example,

> Ed was a suspicious, hallucinating inpatient who frequently irritated other group members by his intrusive, inappropriate behavior. During one session, Frank confronted Ed in a critical manner about an incident on the ward. Ed began to distort some

of Frank's comments and quickly became angry and threatening. My female co-therapist and I tried to calm down the situation, to no avail. When Ed suddenly clenched his fists and stood up, my co-therapist also stood up and suggested that he accompany her out of the group room to "talk things over." After they left, I asked the other patients what they thought of the situation. Frank expressed some remorse for his comments, and everyone else expressed relief that Ed had left and that the situation had not escalated to physical abuse. Gradually, everyone calmed down. About 10 minutes later, my co-therapist returned with Ed. He had received some medication, had walked around the ward with her, and was now more relaxed. We all discussed the episode in terms of it being a distortion of the facts and a misunderstanding. Frank said he was sorry that his remarks came across as being critical, that he really had intended to give Ed some useful feedback. I commented on how important it was for the group to be a safe place where everyone could learn ways to cope with their illness. I then tried to paraphrase Frank's comments in less personal terms. Ed was able to accept this feedback, and the session continued.

A second advantage of a co-therapy approach is that the therapists can model nonpsychotic interactions with one another, and this can be useful for many patients. Sometimes the two leaders are the only people in the room who are able to test reality, and they can play off each other to help a patient challenge the basis behind his or her distorted perception or belief. Helping a patient reality test may be quite difficult for only one therapist to accomplish, especially when there is little support from the other group members.
For example,

During one session on an inpatient unit, my co-therapist was ill, and I decided to lead the group alone. George began talking about his belief that there were several dimensions of reality and that the reality of the group was no more valid than the others. I said that I thought George was using this discussion to avoid confronting his problems, and I asked the other patients what they thought. To my surprise, the other group members agreed with George, and they all began to consider just how many true realities there were. As the discussion progressed, I found myself thinking that maybe the patients had a point! But because the goals of the group did not include engaging in a philosophical discussion, and because I did not have a co-therapist to help me confront the patients' common belief, I decided that a strategic withdrawal was the best course of action. I said that this topic was very interesting but that it did not seem to be dealing with the group members' reasons for being in the hospital. I suggested we move into another topic area, and we gradually began discussing difficulties that the patients were having in relating with other people.

Despite this example, it usually is possible to hold a group session when one therapist is absent due to a vacation or illness, and this constitutes a third advantage of a co-therapy approach. Particularly in outpatient groups, where many of the members are able to test reality and discuss strategies of coping with their symptoms adequately enough to assist the therapist, it is useful to be able to continue the sessions on schedule, even when one of the leaders is gone. The patients appreciate this, and they are able to remember an appointment better if it is on a regular basis than if it frequently is canceled due to therapist absences. Because of the potential for chaotic behavior and lapses in reality testing in groups of schizophrenic patients, peer-led groups rarely are indicated. In contrast to some other group activities (e.g., consciousness-raising groups), therapy groups require the presence of at least one trained professional leader (Kanas and Farrell 1984), and if this cannot be provided in an integrative group, then the session should be canceled.

A final advantage of the co-therapy approach is to help alleviate the stress and potential for burnout that can result from leading groups of severely mentally ill patients. As has been pointed out by others (Frankel 1993; Geczy and Sultenfuss 1995; LeFevre 1994; Takahashi and Washington 1991), these groups can be emotionally exhausting and difficult to control. Therapeutic progress may be restricted due to the severity of patient pathology, and financial rewards may be limited in treatment settings that deal with schizophrenic patients. Under these circumstances, co-therapists can mutually support one another, increase the sense of safety in the group, and provide clinical feedback to each other during chaotic periods. They can share treatment strategies before a session and rehash important issues and interventions after the group ends. Finally, knowing that at least one other professional understands and values this important work can be tremendously sustaining and morale boosting, even during the most frustrating times.

In outpatient groups, the same two therapists generally lead the sessions. In the inpatient setting, however, staff turnover and schedule changes often make it difficult for the same people to commit to being available to the group for every session. On such units, I have found it useful to train a pool of therapists who can fill in for each other depending on availability. These include both permanent ward-based staff (e.g., nurses, social workers, occupational therapists) as well as off-ward staff or trainees (e.g., psychiatrists, psychologists, psychiatric residents). Although some disruption occurs by substituting therapists, this reflects a reality of life on many hospital units and is workable as long as the leaders are well trained, communicate what happened in previous sessions to each other, and try to arrange to have at least one of the therapists from the previous session participate as a co-therapist in the current session. If more than two therapists are available, the extra people can still observe the session behind a one-way mirror or seated outside of the group circle as silent observers. They then are free to participate in any postgroup rehash that takes place, and they would be available to lead the next session because they have observed the current one. Although Sandison (1994) advocated using four therapists to conduct an inpatient schizophrenic group, too many leaders can be confusing and anxiety producing, and I find that two therapists at a time is optimal for a small psychotherapy group.

A male-female co-therapy team is useful, because some patients relate better to a leader who is of one sex or the other. In addition, the leaders can model opposite-sex interactions and viewpoints that may be helpful during gender-related discussions. However, because transference interpretations generally are not made in groups of schizophrenic patients, it is not as critical to have opposite-sex co-therapy teams as it might be in groups involving higher-functioning patients.

The specific professional background of the leaders is relatively unimportant as long as both are familiar with the symptomatology and treatment of schizophrenia and both are trained to lead the group. In academic programs, supervisor-student co-therapy teams provide a good teaching approach as long as the trainee does not defer too much to the teacher and simply become a passive observer. As in any other therapy group, it is important for co-therapists to participate in more or less the same degree in the sessions and to be seen as equally helpful by the patients. This particularly is important in inpatient settings where there is a pool of trained therapists that rotate in and out of the group and in outpatient settings where one of the therapists needs to miss several sessions due to illness or vacation.

Structural Issues

In my review of 46 controlled studies involving therapy groups for schizophrenic patients (Kanas 1993), I isolated a number of structural characteristics that defined key parameters of this treatment activity. In the inpatient setting, more than half of the groups that mentioned frequency and duration met either two or three times per week, generally in sessions lasting for 1 hour. Most of the groups were open to new patients recently admitted to the ward, consisted of both psychotic and nonpsychotic members, were led by one therapist, and averaged between seven and eight patients. In the outpatient setting, half of the groups met on a weekly basis, and the majority had sessions lasting for 1 hour. Half were open and half were closed to new admissions once they began. Most of the groups were composed entirely of schizophrenic patients and were led by one therapist. The majority averaged between 10 and 12 patients.

A number of structural parameters characteristic of integrative groups can be isolated, and some of these are summarized in Table 4–3. Although these have evolved over time as reasonable guidelines, the reader may choose to change some of these parameters based on his or her own clinical situation.

The inpatient groups usually meet three times per week, although if staff availability allows, this could be extended to four or five times. Although when we first started the sessions lasted for 1 hour, they now last 45 minutes, which seems to be a more realistic duration for psychotic inpatients. The groups are open to new admissions who come to the unit, provided that they have schizophrenia or a related condition and that they can tolerate being in the room without experiencing overwhelming anxiety

Table 4-3. Structural issues

Issue	Inpatient groups	Outpatient groups
Sessions per week	3-5	1-2
Duration of session (minutes)	45	60
Boundary	Open	Closed
Patient composition	Schizophrenic	Schizophrenic
Number of therapists	2	2
Enrolled patients	3-8	8-10
Optimal patient average	5-7	6-8

or becoming too disruptive. Two therapists are better than one, as described. If fewer than three patients are present, there is little opportunity for group interaction, and the session is canceled. More than eight patients in the room can be overstimulating and produces a group that is difficult to handle. Ideally, the sessions will average five to seven patients.

The outpatient groups meet once per week, although in some clinic or day treatment settings a semiweekly format might be possible. Schizophrenic outpatients can tolerate 60-minute sessions. The format is closed or slow-open, admitting new members only when discharges or dropouts result in a group that is becoming too small to be optimal. Although one therapist usually can handle a group composed of schizophrenic patients, I prefer a co-therapy approach. The groups begin with 8-10 patients, and this usually results in an average attendance of 6-8 patients per session, which is optimal.

Medications

Most of the patients in the groups receive antipsychotic medications. Clinically, these two treatment modalities act synergistically, with the medications helping the patients organize their thinking, become less anxious, and experience a lessening of their psychotic symptoms, and the group experience helping them to learn strategies of coping with their psychosis and to develop ways of interacting better with other people. Thus, both approaches are necessary in a complete biopsychosocial treatment plan.

Although group leaders who happen to be physicians may prescribe the patients' medications, this is not done during the sessions. In addition, group time is not used for prolonged discussions of dosage and side effects, because this does not serve the primary goals of the group. It should be made clear that the group is a psychotherapeutic activity, not a medication group, and issues involving dose and side effects should be dealt with in other settings. For outpatients, this might be done in a separate clinic by other physicians. Problems with side effects may be addressed individually before or after the session; in acute situations, the patient may need to be escorted out of the room for an individual evaluation.

There are two instances when discussions involving medications are congruent with the goals of the group. One instance would concern a discussion of the value of medications as a coping strategy for dealing with psychotic experiences, particularly if patients are allowed by their physicians temporarily to increase their dose when they feel more anxious or are under increased stress in their lives. In this instance, the patients should be encouraged to share their views on this matter, not just ask for advice from the therapists. In many cases, stable group members may be able to convince more psychotic individuals who refuse medications that these drugs will help them deal with their frightening experiences.

The second instance when a general discussion of medications is useful relates to the patients' feelings about having to take these drugs. By sharing their feelings, a bond may be built up between the group members, resulting in a sense of commonality and increased cohesiveness. This also can lead to the expression of feelings about having to cope with a serious chronic mental illness.

For example,

> In one outpatient group, Harold asked me what I thought about the antipsychotic medication he was on and whether I thought his dose was too high. Irene also asked me if her dose was adjusted correctly, because she was experiencing some side effects:

stiffness in her muscles and blurring of her vision. She wondered if it was worth taking the medication. James also reported blurring of vision and said he was thinking of stopping his medication. He asked me if his dose was right. I responded by saying that the patients should speak with their clinic physician about specific doses, because this really was not the purpose of the group. However, I said that I was struck by the fact that all three of them had concerns about the value of taking medications, and I asked them how they felt about the need to take these potent tranquilizers. Irene admitted that she did not like to take her medications because of their side effects but also because it meant she still had her illness. When I asked Harold and James if they had similar thoughts, they said yes. The discussion then moved on to the topic of the frustration and despair that the patients felt at having a chronic mental illness that was incurable and that seriously impaired their ability to function in everyday life.

Medications are a fact of life for most schizophrenic patients. The group can help them see the value of taking these drugs and of sharing strategies that will help them learn how to use their medications appropriately. Sometimes advice from another patient is much more acceptable than advice from a physician or family members who have not been on antipsychotic medications. This patient-to-patient interaction should generally be encouraged in the group and is especially useful in confronting a resistant member who might distrust feedback from people who have not had the experience of being psychotic.

References

Africa B, Schwartz SR: Schizophrenic disorders, in Review of General Psychiatry, 3rd Edition. Edited by Goldman HH. Norwalk, CT, Appleton & Lange, 1992, pp 198–214

American Psychiatric Association: Schizophrenia and other psychotic disorders, in Diagnostic and Statistical Manual of Mental Disorders, 4th Edition. Washington, DC, American Psychiatric Association, 1994, pp 273–315

Breier A, Strauss JS: Self-control in psychotic disorders. Arch Gen Psychiatry 40:1141–1145, 1983

Cohen CI, Berk LA: Personal coping styles of schizophrenic outpatients. Hosp Community Psychiatry 36:407–410, 1985

Corrigan PW, Storzbach DM: Behavioral interventions for alleviating psychotic symptoms. Hosp Community Psychiatry 44:341–347, 1993

de Bosset F: Group psychotherapy in chronic psychiatric outpatients: a Toronto model. Int J Group Psychother 41:65–78, 1991

Dobson DJG, McDougall G, Busheikin J, et al: Effects of social skills training and social milieu treatment on symptoms of schizophrenia. Psychiatric Services 46:376–380, 1995

Drake RE, Sederer LI: The adverse effects of intensive treatment of chronic schizophrenia. Compr Psychiatry 27:313–326, 1986

Erickson RC: Heterogeneous groups: a legitimate alternative. Group 10:21–26, 1986

Falloon IRH, Talbot RE: Persistent auditory hallucinations: coping mechanisms and implications for management. Psychol Med 11:329–339, 1981

Frankel B: Groups for the chronic mental patient and legacy of failure. Int J Group Psychother 43:157–172, 1993

Geczy B, Sultenfuss J: Group psychotherapy on state hospital admission wards. Int J Group Psychother 45:1–15, 1995

Kanas N: Group psychotherapy with schizophrenia, in Comprehensive Group Psychotherapy. Edited by Kaplan HI, Sadock BJ. Baltimore, MD, Williams & Wilkins, 1993, pp 407–418

Kanas N, Barr MA: Short-term homogeneous group therapy for schizophrenic inpatients: a questionnaire evaluation. Group 6:32–38, 1982

Kanas N, Barr MA: Self-control of psychotic productions in schizophrenics. Arch Gen Psychiatry 41:919–920, 1984

Kanas N, Farrell D: Group psychotherapy, in Review of General Psychiatry. Edited by Goldmann HH. Los Altos, CA, Lange Medical Publications, 1984, pp 540–548

Kanas N, Smith AJ: Schizophrenic group process: a comparison and replication using the HIM-G. Group 14:246–252, 1990

Kanas N, Rogers M, Kreth E, et al: The effectiveness of group psychotherapy during the first three weeks of hospitalization: a controlled study. J Nerv Ment Dis 168:487–492, 1980

Kaplan HI, Sadock BJ (eds): Comprehensive Textbook of Psychiatry, 5th Edition. Baltimore, MD, Williams & Wilkins, 1989

Lazerson JS, Zilbach JJ: Gender issues in group psychotherapy, in Comprehensive Group Psychotherapy, 3rd Edition. Edited by Kaplan HI, Sadock BJ. Baltimore, MD, Williams & Wilkins, 1993, pp 682–693

LeFevre DC: The power of countertransference in groups for the severely mentally ill. Group Analysis 27:441–447, 1994

Leopold HS: Selective group approaches with psychotic patients in hospital settings. Am J Psychother 30:95–102, 1976

MacDonald WS, Blochberger CW, Maynard HM: Group therapy: a comparison of patient-led and staff-led groups on an open hospital ward. Psychiatr Q 38 (suppl):290–303, 1964

MacKenzie KR: Introduction to Time-Limited Group Psychotherapy. Washington, DC, American Psychiatric Press, 1990

MacKenzie KR: Where is here and when is now?: the adaptational challenge of mental health reform for group psychotherapy. Int J Group Psychother 44:407–428, 1994

Misunis RJ, Feist BJ, Thorkelsson JG, et al: Outpatient groups for chronic psychiatric patients. Group 14:111–120, 1990

Pattison EM, Brissenden E, Wohl T: Assessing special effects of inpatient group psychotherapy. Int J Group Psychother 17:283–297, 1967

Sandison R: Working with schizophrenics individually and in groups: understanding the psychotic process. Group Analysis 27:393–406, 1994

Strassberg DS, Roback HB, Anchor KN, et al: Self-disclosure in group therapy with schizophrenics. Arch Gen Psychiatry 32:1259–1261, 1975

Takahashi T, Washington WP: A group-centered object relations approach to group psychotherapy with severely disturbed patients. Int J Group Psychother 41:79–96, 1991

Taylor JR, Strassberg DS: The effects of sex composition on cohesiveness and interpersonal learning in short-term personal growth groups. Psychotherapy 23:267–273, 1986

Weiner MF: Outcome of psychoanalytically oriented group psychotherapy. Group 8:3–12, 1984

World Health Organization: The ICD-10 Classification of Mental and Behavioural Disorders. Geneva, Switzerland, World Health Organization, 1992

Yalom ID: Inpatient Group Psychotherapy. New York, Basic Books, 1983

CHAPTER 5

Clinical Issues:
Treatment Strategies

*I*n the integrative model for treating schizophrenic patients in therapy groups, the therapists use treatment techniques and encourage discussion topics that are congruent with the group goals and the needs of the patients. The importance of confidentiality and patient safety are stressed. Typical group sessions progress from first identifying a problematic issue for discussion (e.g., auditory hallucinations), to then generalizing this topic to all of the members, and finally, to encouraging the members to share strategies that will help them cope with the problem. Special issues relate to beginning and ending the groups, adding new members and saying goodbye to departing members, and orienting patients to the group before they begin their first session.

Therapist Stance

In leading a group of schizophrenic patients, the therapists behave differently from the way they might behave in a group of higher-functioning individuals. This is due to the goals of the group and the needs of the patients. Some characteristics of the proper therapist stance are shown in Table 5–1.

Because the members often are disorganized and distracted by hallucinations and other psychotic experiences, they may tune

Table 5–1.　Therapist stance

Active and directive in keeping group members focused on the topic

Clear, consistent, and concrete with interventions

Supportive and diplomatic with comments

Open and willing to give opinions and advice that are appropriate to the discussion

Here-and-now (rather than there-and-then) focused

Encouraging of patient-to-patient (rather than patient-to-therapist) interactions

out the external environment or respond to internal stimulation in inappropriate ways. Consequently, the therapists need to be active and directive in keeping them focused on the discussion topic. Kibel (1991) likened this role of the therapist to that of a symphony conductor who must orchestrate his or her own special group. This particularly is important in the inpatient setting, because the members are more acutely ill. However, outpatient therapists also need to keep the group on track. For example,

> In one outpatient group, Alan began the session by declaring that he recently had been told that he had emphysema. As he spoke, it became apparent that his case was quite mild and that it was not of great concern to him. Nevertheless, this led several patients to relate various physical problems that they had and to discuss the medications they were taking. Brenda asked me for my advice about a medicine, and I briefly answered her. When the patients continued to discuss medical problems, I became concerned that too much time was being used in this area, which was not related to the group goals. Although I wondered if this discussion was a way to avoid talking about more personal issues, I decided that it would be more prudent to make a general observational comment rather than to make an interpretation about intent. I stated that we had been spending a lot of time talking about physical problems and wondered about what kind of mental problems people had been having. After a brief pause, Alan described having difficulties with racing thoughts, and several other patients stated that they too had trouble organizing their ideas. This led to a general discussion about how to cope

with disorganized thoughts and the ways in which this condition interfered with their lives.

Interventions need to be clear, consistent, and concrete to be understood by patients who are psychotic or sleepy from their medications, and it is useful to repeat important points. At the same time, interventions should be supportive in style to minimize the probability of a patient taking offense or hearing the message through a persecutory distortion. For example, when interrupting a member who is introducing an extraneous topic into the discussion, the therapist can make it clear that what the patient is saying is interesting but that it is not quite on the topic, and that perhaps it can be discussed another time. Other supportive comments include praising a quiet patient who begins to speak, acknowledging the return of a member who left the room temporarily, and giving positive reinforcement to a patient who pays a compliment to another member of the group.

Because transference rarely is interpreted in schizophrenic groups, and because the therapist role includes modeling nonpsychotic thinking, it is permissible for the leaders occasionally to give advice and offer their personal opinions about a matter if this will advance the group discussion and assist with reality testing. Obviously, such comments are not made for self-aggrandizement or for reasons unrelated to the group members' needs. The therapists need to guard against making too many advice-giving comments, however, because their value for patients has been questioned (Kanas and Barr 1982) and because they may encourage patient-to-therapist interactions rather than patient-to-patient interactions. In addition, discussions that focus on the immediate experiences of the members during the sessions (the here and now) tend to be more powerful and productive of change than discussions that deal with issues from the patients' past (the there and then). A therapy group is a unique environment that allows the members to learn from each other, and it is useful for the therapists to encourage this and to save their expert advice for after the session.

There are a number of ways that a group leader can encourage the members to interact with one each other. For example, one way is to state that because a patient really is talking about another patient, he should look at her and make his comments directly to her. Alternatively, by looking away or pointing to another group member, a therapist can redirect a patient who continually addresses the therapist onto a more appropriate individual. If patients persist in making their comments to the leader, then this might be an appropriate issue for discussion. This emphasis on patients interacting with and learning from each other distinguishes therapy groups from educational or advice-giving activities (e.g., medication or current events groups).

Patient Safety

A therapy group for schizophrenic patients must be a safe environment where the members can discuss their problems with a minimum of anxiety and conflict. When too much tension exists, it may activate murderous fantasies or fears of losing control, and patients may regress or become more psychotic. The therapists can contribute to a safe environment by making supportive comments, by steering the discussion away from an anxiety-producing topic to one that is less emotionally arousing, by abstracting and depersonalizing an issue, and by taking steps to reduce interpersonal anger. Sometimes they must be explicit in stating that the group feels unsafe and that a change in subject is warranted. At other times, a more diplomatic approach is necessary.

For example,

Charles was a new patient in an inpatient group who stated that he believed he was Christ. One of the other patients, Daniel, became agitated and blurted out that *he* was Christ! Charles then clarified that he was the Servant of God. Because neither patient seemed ready to have their grandiose delusions challenged, and because both were becoming increasingly anxious and defensive, I became concerned that the situation might escalate into a physical confrontation or a psychological decompensation. I thought it best to defuse the issue diplomatically. I asked Charles if being the Servant of God wasn't really like being an apostle of Christ, and he said yes. This seemed to mollify Daniel, because he could continue with his belief that he was Christ without having to compete with Charles. The situation quickly de-escalated, with both patients continuing to have a special religious role. Their delusions would be challenged in a future group after their antipsychotic medications had taken effect and after each patient was better able to test the reality of his belief.

One possible indicator of anxiety occurs when a patient requests to leave the room. This particularly occurs in inpatient groups, where the patients are more fragile and intolerant of group tension. The usual excuse is having to go to the bathroom. When patients want to leave, the therapists should always confront them, asking why they are leaving and suggesting that the departure may be related to a disturbing issue in the group. They also are encouraged to stay until the session ends. If they cannot, they are asked to return as soon as possible. If they do return, they should be praised for coming back. If departures become frequent, this becomes an issue for discussion.

For example,

During a session on an inpatient unit, Erik suddenly got up and started to leave the room. I asked him where he was going, and he said that he had to go to the bathroom. I asked him if the group was making him nervous, and he said no, that he just needed to use the bathroom. I told him to go ahead but to please return to the group. He left and returned about 20 minutes later. At the first break in the ongoing group discussion, I briefly acknowledged Erik's return and said that I was glad that he came back. Near the end of the next session, Erik again got up to go to the bathroom. I asked him if he couldn't wait for 15 more minutes until the group ended, but he said no. He did not return to the group. At the beginning of the following session, I asked Erik if his leaving the room during the previous two sessions was because it was hard for him to be in the group. This time he admitted that he became nervous being in a room with other people, and he said that his voices told him to leave and go outside where it was safer. I asked some of the other patients to comment, and they said that the group seemed safe to them and that Erik should try to remain in the room for the entire session. I reinforced this and asked Erik to please tell us whenever the discussion made him anxious or the voices started to tell him to leave. He said he would. He also was able to remain in the room for the entire session.

Because many schizophrenic patients are extremely vigilant and suspicious, the therapists can reduce their suspicions and make them feel safer by stressing issues of confidentiality. The members should be warned against discussing what transpires in the group with people on the outside. The therapists should be explicit about what type of charting they do and who has access to the medical records. Students and staff who observe the group through a one-way mirror or who sit in the room outside of the group circle should introduce themselves prior to the beginning of each session, and the reasons for their presence should be explained. People should not be allowed to observe if they come late and have not introduced themselves. Observers should be told not to discuss the group content with friends and acquaintances. If the group is videotaped, written informed consent is mandatory, and videotapes need to be carefully controlled. Provided that the above steps are taken, an environment of trust can be established in a schizophrenic group, and sessions can be observed by others with minimal impact on the group process.

Discussion Topics

Importance of Patient Condition and Group Duration

Because the goals of a therapy group for schizophrenic patients include coping with symptoms and improving interpersonal relationships, the issues that are discussed in the sessions should be congruent with these goals. However, the topics vary somewhat depending on whether the group is composed of the acutely psychotic patients generally found on an inpatient unit or the more stable chronic patients found in clinics and day treatment programs. The types of topics discussed also depend on whether the session is occurring early or late in the group's life.

In groups of acutely ill patients or early in the life of the group, typical issues that are discussed include auditory hallucinations; persecutory, referential, and grandiose delusions; thought insertion and thought broadcasting; loose associations or other types of disorganized thinking; and problems interacting with other people. In addition, the patients can discuss "safe" emotions that are related to the above topics, such as depression or hopelessness over their condition. Emotional topics that produce anxiety (e.g., anger at someone in the group, issues involving conflicts in sexual orientation or identity) should be avoided, because they can cause schizophrenic patients to regress and become more symptomatic, as will be discussed later. The focus generally is practical and relates to problems that the patients are having at the present time. During the first session or whenever a new patient is admitted to the group, topics that are appropriate for discussion are mentioned in nonclinical terms to avoid misunderstanding and to keep the group focused on concrete issues. For example, the word *paranoid* means different things to different patients (e.g., suspicious, cautious, crazy, worried); to be clear, the therapists will ask them what they mean in everyday terms whenever they use this or some other clinical term. (The word *schizophrenia* is usually translated as *nervous breakdown* by the therapists.) Patients starting an open inpatient group frequently are given the direction that: "In this group, we usually talk about hearing voices, feeling suspicious, being confused, or having problems relating with others." This sets the tone and prompts the patients to think in clear terms about their present symptoms and ways to cope with them.

For patients who are less psychotic and more stable or who have been together in a group for some time, these topics still may be relevant if they have not been thoroughly discussed. However, the focus usually takes on a more longitudinal perspective as the members discuss current problems in reference to long-standing maladaptive patterns of behavior or chronic aspects of their disease. In addition, the topics may be more sophisticated. For example, chronic patients in outpatient groups are able to deal with issues related to how their long-standing distrust of others has made them isolative or how their poor social skills have led them to make naive mistakes, such as loaning out money to "friends" that was never returned. They also can tolerate emotional and anxiety-producing issues better than acute patients, such as despair over having a chronic mental illness or anger at people who have caused them difficulties in their lives. However, care still needs to be exercised around issues that raise too much anxiety.

Examples of Helpful Discussion Topics

Hallucinations. Topics related to auditory hallucinations are commonly discussed in the group. Less typically considered are visual and other types of hallucinations. Some patients are able to test the reality of these experiences, and others are not. Usually the former have a modicum of reality sense so that they can step outside the experience and examine it as being ego-alien. Consensual validation from the other group members in the here and now can help a patient determine the reality basis of a hallucination. Note that the experience itself is perceived as real by the patient even though he or she is able to admit that it is internally generated and part of the illness. Once a patient admits that a hallucination is foreign, he or she can then learn ways to test the reality of similar experiences and discuss ways to cope with them.

For example,

> In one short-term outpatient group, I noticed that Fred was talk-ing to himself. I asked him if he was responding to voices, and he said yes. I asked the other patients if they had heard anyone talking to Fred, and several said no. I then asked them to give Fred some feedback on his voices. Gloria said that she had no-ticed Fred talking to himself in other sessions, and she told him that his experiences were all in his mind. Henry said that he also had heard voices in the past but that they had largely gone away since he had begun taking medications. Irving said that his voices got quieter when he engaged in some activity that occupied his attention, such as watching television or reading a magazine. Joe said that his voices went away when he spoke with someone else. I asked Fred what he thought about this feedback, and he admitted that the voices he heard probably did not come from real people even though he clearly perceived what he thought was external speech. I stated that it was important to "check out" the reality of such experiences with his therapist or a trusted friend. I also asked him what he thought of the coping strategies suggested by the other patients in the group. He said that he thought that some of them would be useful for him, and he would try them out when his voices became "too loud."

Delusions.   Persecutory, referential, and grandiose delusions are the most common types of distorted belief experienced by schizo-phrenic patients. Patients who are able to test the reality of their delusions with the help of the group are ready to discuss useful coping strategies. Unlike hallucinations, however, which can be challenged in the here and now by the other group members, distorted beliefs are more difficult to address because they pertain to an individual's personal way of thinking about the world. Members who have had delusions in the past but have been able to give them up with the help of medication and therapy are in the best position to give helpful feedback to newer patients still trapped in a distorted belief system. For example,

> During one session on an acute-care inpatient unit, Kevin admitted to having a belief that the food was poisoned. I asked the other patients what they thought of the ward food. Leonard said that he once believed that someone wanted to poison his food, but that he changed his mind after being on antipsychotic medications and discussing his belief with members of the staff. Mike said that he felt the ward food was fine. When no one further responded, I went around the group circle and asked all of the other patients for their opinion. At the end of this go-around, it became obvious that no one but Kevin believed that the ward food was poisoned. I then asked the members to give Kevin feedback about his belief, and several told him that he was wrong and that he should eat the food without fear. Kevin said that he would think about it. During the next 2 days he began to eat again, and in the subsequent group session, I and several of the patients gave him some positive feedback for this behavioral change. He admitted that the food seemed alright.

Some patients believe that thoughts are being placed in their minds (thought insertion) or believe that they can project their thoughts to other people (thought broadcasting). When on the receiving end, the thoughts may be experienced as being those of someone else. Many patients can give a good reason why this is happening to them, and they invoke some form of telepathy as the mechanism of action. They cite the work of parapsychologists or stories in the popular press as justification for their experience. It is important not to engage in a debate about the reality of telepathy with these patients, because it occupies a great deal of group time and usually resolves nothing. Rather, the therapist can point out how the experience interferes with the patient's life in a negative manner.

For example,

> During an inpatient group session, several members were discussing their auditory hallucinations. Norma volunteered that she did not hear voices but that she was in constant communi-

cation with her boyfriend via telepathy. She stated that he would transmit his thoughts to her and that she had the ability to respond back to him in return. Their conversation generally consisted of sexual content and their desire to see one another when she was released from the hospital. When Olive challenged the reality of these experiences, Norma stated that telepathy was a fact because she had seen people on television state that they had similar telepathic experiences. I asked Norma how her experiences affected her life. She admitted that her family and friends did not believe her and thought that she was "schizophrenic." Furthermore, they brought her to the hospital when she became disruptive and out of control at home. At my suggestion, some of the group members gave Norma advice about ways she could control her behavior and be less intrusive and angry in expressing her beliefs. In a later session, Norma admitted to having persecutory and referential ideation, and this also was seen as a cause for her behavioral and interpersonal problems.

Challenging a delusion is not always successful, especially if the patient cannot test reality well enough to examine his or her belief system. Sometimes a strategic retreat to another topic or another patient is necessary. At other times, a delusion can be confronted through a dramatic action.

For example,

Paul was a delusional patient on an inpatient unit who continually expressed a belief that there was a plot to kill him. When I asked him about this, he mentioned that there was a poster on the ward that indicated his imminent death. Because no one in the room knew about this poster, I asked everyone to join him in looking at it. We all got up, left the group room, and went to the day room. On one of the walls was an antinuclear power poster that pictured an atomic explosion with a dead bird among some ruins. Below this was a nuclear reactor with a skull and crossbones on it. Written on the poster were the words: "This could happen to you!" After returning to the group room, I offered my opinion that the poster was warning of the dangers of a nuclear accident and did not refer to any plot to kill Paul. He did not believe this explanation. I then asked the other patients for their opinion. Several agreed with me. Paul continued to be skeptical, and I asked him to give this feedback some thought. Over the next few days, he began to question this belief and other thoughts related to his fear of imminent danger.

Disorganized thinking. Discussions involving loose associations and other forms of disorganized thinking are both difficult
and easy to work with. They are difficult because they involve an
abstract concept: the process of thinking, rather than a perception
(e.g., hallucination) or a belief (e.g., delusion). Consequently,
some patients have difficulty realizing that their thinking is disorganized when compared with other people. However, the discussion is made easier when a patient demonstrates his or her
disorganization during the session for all to see and to comment
on in the here and now.

For example,

> During one inpatient group, Quincy repeatedly had problems
> staying on the subject. I asked the other members if they could
> understand him, and several said no. I told Quincy that I also
> had problems following his ideas because after he had expressed
> one thought, this would lead to another idea that was off the
> track. I suggested that he try to stop talking as soon as he made
> his point. I also asked him if it would be alright if we gave him
> feedback as soon as he started drifting so that he could learn
> when he was beginning to confuse us. He said that would be
> fine. During the rest of the session, I verbally interrupted Quincy
> whenever he started to become loose or tangential, while I also
> tried to paraphrase his main idea. He responded well to this feed-
> back. Over the next several sessions, he made comments during
> the discussions that were shorter and more congruent with the
> ideas that were being expressed.

It is useful for disorganized patients to receive immediate
feedback when their ideas begin to wander. Hopefully, this experience will help them learn to self-regulate and keep their utter-
ances succinct and understandable by others, both inside and
outside of the group.

Relations with others. Because most schizophrenic patients are
isolated individuals, and because group therapy is by nature an
interpersonal treatment modality, discussions concerning the improvement of relations with others are common in the groups,
especially as the patients become less psychotic and more interested in exploring their maladaptive interactions. Although a few
patients deny wanting to relate more successfully with other peo-

ple, I believe that these people are responding from fear and mistrust, because they do open up in the group as they become more comfortable with the other members. For some patients, simply learning ways to make contact with someone else is a valuable experience.
For example,

In one outpatient group, Rodney, a quiet, withdrawn individual, began talking about a fast-food restaurant that he liked that was near his apartment. Sam mentioned another place nearby that was much cheaper. Rodney began asking him questions about the place. Tanya also became interested, saying that she needed to save money. As he talked, Sam began to praise the restaurant not only as a place to eat inexpensively, but also as a place where the workers and clientele seemed friendly. To illustrate this point, he stated that he liked to go to the restaurant every Sunday for breakfast, and he began to notice another man there who had a similar schedule. They gradually began talking to one another and found that they had things in common. Now he looks forward to seeing this person whenever he goes to the restaurant. I commented that for Sam, this restaurant had great value, not only financially but also socially. I further stated that one can meet people anywhere, and that all that is needed is a common interest and someone willing to break the ice. Both Sam and Tanya agreed. I asked Rodney if he had spoken with anyone at his restaurant, and he said no. The group discussion then moved into the area of giving Rodney advice about how he could meet people in everyday situations.

Other patients have difficulty becoming close and intimate. Superficially, they can make contact, but they cannot take the risks necessary to turn a contact into a friendship. Discussions related to this issue can be quite rewarding, not only for a given patient but for the other group members as well.
For example,

Victor was a man in his early 20s who was in a long-term outpatient group for schizophrenic patients. He had long-standing difficulties relating with other people, especially women. In the group, he was able to talk about his shyness and admitted that he had never gone out on a date with a woman. During one session, he stated that he was thinking of asking out a female acquaintance who was in his sheltered workshop. Several of the women in the group encouraged him to do this, especially Ursula, a schizoaffective woman in her early 40s. Over the course of the next few sessions, Ursula continued to coach Victor about his plans. She gave him very specific advice, such as how to ask a woman out on a date and how to behave the first time. In a subsequent session, Victor began the group by proudly announcing that he had indeed asked the woman out for a 30-minute coffee date and that all had gone well. The group responded to the news with much excitement and joy, and Ursula especially was happy and enthusiastic to hear the details. This modest beginning in interpersonal relatedness greatly improved Victor's confidence and self-esteem. It also had an important effect on Ursula, because she seemed pleased that she could help someone and that her advice really meant something. In addition, the group became more cohesive and energized as a result of this experience.

In groups of stable patients who have been meeting for some time, long-term maladaptive patterns of relating with other people can be discussed. These members are ready to take an historical perspective concerning their relationship difficulties and to see that their problems are more chronic in nature, not simply related to the acute exacerbations of their illness.

For example,

In one outpatient group, Walter related his current problems in interacting with others to his long-term fears of intimacy. He admitted to never having learned how to engage other people, and he said that he had made few friends in his life. Xavier said that his problem was not really knowing how to trust others, and he always believed that people who got too close to him could be dangerous. Zeke said that he tried to make friends in the past, but that people seemed to take advantage of him. He described several episodes where he had naively lent money to acquaintances but had never been repaid. Yolanda said that she had no problem making friends, but that they also seemed to take advantage of her. I commented that making friends could be risky, but that the alternative was a life of isolation and loneliness. I pointed out that some of the group members never seemed to have learned how to form long-term relationships and that being too suspicious or too naively trusting could lead to interpersonal problems. This led to a discussion about ways to meet people, evaluate their intentions, seek common interests, and encourage a new contact to evolve gradually into a friendship.

Interpersonal skills are improved not only by the discussion itself but also by the group interaction accompanying this discussion. By relating with one another during the sessions, patients learn to trust other people and practice interpersonal skills that can be transferred to situations outside of the group. In a sense, almost any discussion topic is useful if patients actively discuss it with one another. For this reason, therapists should take a strongly interpersonal stance in a group of schizophrenic patients by encouraging them to talk to one another and give each other feedback about how they are coming across during the sessions. In inpatient settings, group members may be encouraged to spend time together on the ward to continue their relationships. In outpatient settings, they are encouraged to practice interpersonal lessons learned in the group with family and friends on the outside, then report back on how things went.

Emotions.   Discussions about emotions can bond patients together and help them feel understood by others. Especially productive are feelings related to the vicissitudes of schizophrenia, such as loneliness over isolation from others and depression and despair over having a chronic illness. As they talk about their feelings, the patients sometimes ventilate them as well, and this can be useful as long as the experience is not overwhelming. In some cases, emotional issues foster friendships in the group.
For example,

> During one inpatient session, Arthur, a relatively stable patient who was about to be discharged, began talking about his loneliness. He described being withdrawn from people during the past 9 years since his first breakdown. In response, Ben described his own feelings of loneliness and related them to the isolation he felt while growing up in a large family. The therapist commented on how much these two patients had in common and suggested that perhaps they could continue their relationship on the ward or even after they were discharged. As the session ended and the patients began to walk out of the room, Ben gently patted Arthur on the shoulder, a nonverbal indicator of the support and commonality these two men felt for one another.

Issues involving despair are surprisingly well tolerated by schizophrenic patients, especially outpatients in therapy groups that have been meeting for awhile. Discussions concerning the despair that these patients feel about having a chronic mental illness seem to bond them together. These discussions usually are quite animated, with the group members making good eye contact and participating at an active level. For example,

> In one outpatient group, several patients were talking about a number of problems they had that were related to reality testing and interpersonal relationships. Because the discussion seemed to be focusing on the sequelae of their schizophrenia, I commented that it must be difficult for them to deal with having a chronic mental illness. Colin said that it was difficult, especially because it affected his relations with his family. Darlene said that she sometimes felt depressed when she considered being this way for the rest of her life. Other patients described having feelings of despair over their condition. I noticed that all the patients were involved with this discussion, spontaneously interacting and making good eye contact. The members seemed to gather strength in realizing that they were not alone in having problems related to their illness. Many of the comments were supportive and addressed positive coping strategies. I needed to intervene only occasionally, because the patients were carrying the bulk of the discussion themselves. The session ended more optimistically than it began, with the members becoming more cohesive and aware of the common bond they shared.

Advice giving.   Although, as mentioned earlier, repeated therapist-to-patient advice giving is not an ideal use of group time, it can be helpful in limited situations. For example, a brief review of medication side effects can lead to a discussion about how it feels to be on antipsychotic drugs for a chronic illness. Similarly, for patients who are ready to leave the hospital, a brief statement describing halfway houses can alleviate anxiety and result in a discussion about the pain of being discharged from the ward (and the group). Therapists should encourage the patients to give each other advice, because it is more experientially relevant than when it comes from the therapists, and because it encourages the patients to interact with one another. Advice giving takes on more importance in outpatient than in inpatient groups, because the members are quite interested in issues related to living arrangements, jobs, education, and so on, and because they have less opportunity to share information with each other during the week than do members of an inpatient group.

Examples of Harmful
Discussion Topics

Anxiety-producing issues.   Some topic areas can be harmful for patients in a schizophrenic group. For example, topics that raise the anxiety level to intolerable degrees can produce regression in these patients, especially if the topics are accompanied by anger and verbal aggression between members of the group. Many schizophrenic patients have murderous fantasies and fears of losing control, and anger is quite threatening to them. Acute inpatients are more vulnerable than outpatients, but even the latter can react poorly to interpersonal anger.

For example,

> In one long-term outpatient group, Ester got angry at Fern for not agreeing more with her in the group, particularly because they were the only two women. During her outburst, the other patients (all men) remained silent. The two therapists both commented on the anger and moved the discussion onto a safer topic. At the next session a week later, Fern did not attend. Several of the male patients began talking about times in their lives when they felt vulnerable and unsafe, and the therapists related this theme to the previous session. The men admitted that Ester's anger at Fern had frightened them, and they expressed the fear that she would become angry at them. They proceeded to discuss how difficult it was for them to deal with anger and the fear that they would lose control and hurt someone or possibly decompensate. The therapists pointed out that this did not happen during the previous week. The session concluded with the patients agreeing that anger could be discussed in the group, but that the therapists would intervene if it became too intense or if the group environment became unsafe.

Sexual material also can be poorly tolerated by psychotic patients. For those with conflicts involving sexual orientation or identity, discussions about sex can make them quite anxious and lead to decompensation. For others who are homosexual but have not revealed this fact in the group, it raises the dilemma of whether and when to come out with this information. For still others who have bizarre sexual delusions, these discussions can feed right into these beliefs. For example,

In one inpatient group, Gary became quite disturbed when several of the male patients began talking about having sex with women. In his psychotic state, he had serious gender-identity problems with which he barely was able to cope. As the discussion progressed, Gary became agitated and expressed the idea that he was both a man and a woman, with male sexual characteristics above the waist and female genitalia below. His thinking became progressively more disorganized, and he stood up in a threatening manner. He had to be escorted out of the group and subsequently received additional medication.

Unconscious conflicts and transference. Issues that reveal unconscious conflicts through uncovering techniques and the interpretation of transference can produce intolerable anxiety in psychotic patients and lead to a worsening of symptoms (Drake and Sederer 1986; Geczy and Sultenfuss 1995; Kanas et al. 1980; MacDonald et al. 1964; Pattison et al. 1967; Strassberg et al. 1975; Weiner 1984). In a sense, schizophrenic patients are struggling to produce order out of chaos and to deal with autistic and primary process thinking. Opening them up psychologically can be countertherapeutic, especially for acutely psychotic inpatients. This is not to say that they cannot achieve some understanding of coping strategies and maladaptive relationships, but generally insight in a psychodynamic sense is not a safe, therapeutic goal in groups composed of schizophrenic patients.

Ways to Develop Topics

Discussions involving relevant topic areas can be encouraged in several ways. Therapists can explicitly mention examples of issues that are appropriate for the group, and this generally occurs in the first session or whenever a new member is added. If patients stray into a nonproductive area, they can gently be reminded that they are deviating from the topic and be asked to go back to the original theme. Some discussions need to be reframed into a more relevant area. For example, concern about a medication side effect may be restructured into a discussion of feelings about having to take drugs for a chronic mental illness. Therapists must be mindful about keeping the group on track and keeping it focused on issues related to the group goals.

Two specific techniques help develop a topic during the course of a session. The first consists of raising an issue in nonpersonal, general terms initially, then asking the members to consider it in more personal, specific terms that relate to them. For example, if patients are reluctant to talk about their persecutory delusions, a therapist can begin by briefly discussing how some people with nervous breakdowns feel inappropriately threatened by others and how this gets them into trouble. The therapist then can ask them if they have ever felt suspicious in ways that later were shown to be unwarranted. Going from general to specific helps the patients participate in a discussion without feeling threatened. It also helps them see that they are not alone in having psychotic experiences.

The second technique is to identify a topic area, then ask each member to comment on it in a go-around. In this manner, all of the members must comment on the issue and relate it to themselves, if only to deny having any problems with it. After all of the members have had a chance to give their perspective on a topic, they then can share coping strategies. In some sessions, only one topic will be discussed, whereas in others there will be time for two or even three areas to be considered.

Coping Strategies

The integrative group therapy model encourages the members to share strategies of coping with their symptoms. For the vast majority of patients who are bothered by psychotic symptoms, these become the primary focus. Ways of improving reality testing ability and lessening the impact of hallucinations and delusions are quite amenable to psychosocial interventions (Breier and Strauss 1983; Cohen and Berk 1985; Corrigan and Storzbach 1993; Dobson et al. 1995; Falloon and Talbot 1981; Kanas and Barr 1984). In addition, the group is useful for helping acute patients present their thoughts in a more organized manner. For those patients who suffer primarily from negative symptoms or interpersonal problems, the group can help them become less withdrawn, more verbal, and more interactive through their participation in the sessions. Coping strategies vary, but certain patterns emerge. Some patients find that they experience more psychotic symptoms and relationship problems when they are under stress or in an anxiety-producing situation. For them, reducing stressful stimulation helps, such as being alone, taking additional medication to relax, playing quiet music, or leaving a chaotic situation. Other patients find that being isolated and understimulated makes their voices seem louder or their persecutory delusions more threatening. For them, increasing their activity level is the key, such as engaging in a hobby, going to a movie, calling a friend, or playing loud music. A significant minority of patients report that going to an isolated area and screaming at their voices to go away sometimes brings them temporary relief. Whatever the strategy, if it works, patients feel a sense of control and mastery over their illness, and this serves to increase hope and decrease despair.

Patients who have evolved relatively successful coping strategies over the years may be encouraged by the therapists to share their experiences with more acutely psychotic patients and with those having difficulty with their symptoms and relationships. In this way, the latter learn helpful strategies and ideas, and the former increase their self-esteem by being helpful and by realizing that they have improved and are better off than others in the group. Some of the coping strategies that are expressed can be quite creative and novel. Consequently, patient-to-patient advice is much more useful than therapist-to-patient advice, and it should be encouraged whenever possible.

Intrasession Sequence

Table 5–2 shows the sequence of events that should occur in a typical session. Ideally, a patient will bring up an appropriate problem area for discussion early in the session (e.g., hearing voices). Other patients then will relate this problem to their own situation (e.g., what the voices are like and how they affect their lives). Although one or two members may deny having the problem, the majority will probably see it as an important issue. Finally, the patients will share coping strategies with one another (e.g., how listening to quiet music or engaging in a hobby will make the voices go away or lessen in intensity). This discussion sequence of identification then generalization then coping allows patients to leave the session feeling that they are not alone with the problem, that they have been able to express themselves in a supportive environment, that they have learned ways of coping with their symptoms, and that they do have some control over their illness. If there is insufficient time to discuss relevant coping strategies, these can be discussed during the next session.

In practice, this sequence seldom occurs spontaneously, because some patients are quiet or guarded and others are anxious or disorganized. When the discussion stalls or rambles, the therapists should intervene to help the members pick a topic and stay on track while discussing it. They may need to reiterate what sorts of topics are relevant for discussion in the group, and they should encourage the patients to speak to and look at each other. When a patient introduces an inappropriate issue, one of the therapists can gently bring the discussion back to the topic with a supportive comment like: "You are bringing up an interesting point, but we were talking about voices, and we should get back to this topic. Maybe we can talk about your issue another time." If the discussion becomes really chaotic or anxiety producing, the therapists should intervene more vigorously to shape the conversation. The more the therapists intervene, the more structured the group becomes, with a resultant decrease in anxiety and a sense that someone is in control.

Table 5–2.   Sequence of events in a typical session

Identification: An appropriate topic that is related to the group goals and the needs of schizophrenic patients should be identified early in the session.

THEN

Generalization: All of the patients should be given the opportunity of discussing the topic as it applies to them—if not done spontaneously, a formal go-around may be useful.

THEN

Coping: The patients should share strategies of coping with the problem with each other, not simply receive advice from the therapists.

Whenever the members succeed in interacting around an appropriate topic, the therapists should be quiet. This allows the patients to practice spontaneous interactions with other members of the group and helps them feel a sense of mastery and control. This can be quite therapeutic, and sometimes a therapist will allow this type of discussion to continue even though the topic area is not ideal. For example, a lively, animated discussion about a television show might be allowed to continue for awhile if the therapists see that the patients are involved and relating well to one another.

In general, the therapists should take their cues from the process of the group, either intervening or holding back depending on the relevance of the topic, the amount of anxiety or conflict present, and the degree to which the patients are spontaneously interacting with one another.

Most sessions consist of open discussions where the patients are encouraged to initiate the conversation and settle on a topic for the day. Although the therapists try to steer the discussion into an appropriate area, little use is made of the formal structured exercises employed by others (Douglas and Mueser 1990; Hierholzer and Liberman 1986; Yalom 1983). However, some sessions allow time for patient orientations and terminations. These are the first and last sessions of a group and sessions that must deal with a new or departing member.

First and Last Sessions

During the first session of a new schizophrenic group, the therapists usually begin by going around the room and asking everyone to state their names. After this is done, the therapists describe the group goals and rules. The patients are told that the group is for people who have had nervous breakdowns and that the goals will be to help them cope with problems such as hearing voices, feeling suspicious, having confused thoughts, and relating poorly with other people. They further are told that the therapists will do all they can to make the group a safe place and that they can expect to learn a great deal by discussing their problems openly with each other. Finally, they are told to come on time; to participate as much as possible in the discussions; and to refrain from loud yelling, physical threats, and hitting the furniture or each other. Next, there should be a go-around where the patients repeat their names, describe their major problems, and say what they hope to get out of the group experience. As problems are described, the therapists try to reframe them in terms of the group goals and the major discussion topics. After this go-around, the therapists select one of the problem areas that seems to affect the most patients and then ask the members to share coping strategies.

Patients are reminded of a group's termination several weeks before the actual date to give them an opportunity to express their thoughts and feelings about this event. During the last session, the therapists acknowledge the end and ask the patients how they feel. It is useful to do a go-around and ask the patients what they got out of their group experience. While this is being done, they can be given feedback about the progress they have made by either the therapists or by other group members. It is important for the last session to be uplifting and positive. At the end, good-byes are said, and the therapists wish the patients well.

New and Departing Members

In ongoing open inpatient groups and long-term outpatient groups, new members are added from time to time. For inpatients, this can occur quite frequently, particularly on acute-care units that have a rapid patient turnover. It is important to integrate the new members quickly because they may attend only a few sessions before being discharged.

In both inpatient and outpatient settings, a simple orientation format is used. First, new patients are introduced to the other members at the beginning of the session. The continuing members then are asked to state the types of issues that are discussed in the group, and the new members are asked which of these represent problems for them. As these are described, the therapists relate them to similar difficulties that the continuing patients have so that the new members can see that they are not alone with their problems. One of these may become the topic for the session. Thus, within 5–10 minutes, new patients are speaking about psychotic or interpersonal issues, they are seeing that they are not alone in having these problems, they are becoming integrated into the group, and a topic is selected for the day's discussion. For example,

> During a session of an inpatient group on an acute-care unit, Hank was attending his first session. I acknowledged this, and we did a go-around where we all introduced ourselves. I then asked the other patients if they could tell Hank what we talked about in this group. They were able to recall three of the topics that I like to reinforce in inpatient groups: hearing voices, feeling suspicious, and relating better with others. I volunteered the fourth: having confused thoughts. I then asked Hank which of these issues represented problems for him. After he said that he heard voices, I asked him to describe what the voices said and how the experience affected his life. I then said that other members of the group had heard voices, and I asked the patients to comment. All but one admitted to hearing voices, and this became the topic for the session.

Patients who are being discharged from inpatient or outpatient groups are given time near the end of their last session to describe their plans and to say what they have gotten out of their experience. The therapists encourage all the members to say goodbye and to voice their support for the departing member. This provides closure and permits the patients to practice appropriate behavior related to termination and loss. It also allows the departing members to see how much they have progressed and instills hope in the patients who remain.

For most outpatients, termination represents a plateau where they will have achieved maximal therapeutic benefit from their group experience. They should be told to give their new learning a try for awhile before considering another group. Because most of the patients will continue to be followed for counseling and medications in an outpatient clinic, they can reapply for another group experience after a few months if they so desire. I have found that time-limited, 12-session outpatient groups can be useful and that more than half of the patients who participate in such a group will choose to join a second "repeater's group" within 2 years if given the opportunity (Kanas 1991; Kanas and Smith 1990). This represents a viable alternative to a continuous long-term outpatient group in settings that do not have the staff resources to commit to such an ongoing treatment modality.

In both inpatient and outpatient settings, another type of termination issue occurs when a member kills him- or herself or becomes worse and has to leave the group. When this happens, many of the remaining members become concerned that the same fate will befall them, and they wonder if the therapists have control of the group. Similarly, the therapists sometimes blame themselves and worry about the impact on the remaining patients. Dramatic events like these need to be openly discussed, and the members should be reassured that the sessions will continue, that the therapists are in control, and that the event that transpired does not necessarily mean that the same thing will happen to any other members of the group.

Pregroup Orientation

In both inpatient and outpatient groups, new members need to be oriented by one of the leaders prior to their first session. This preparation reduces patient anxiety, establishes a working alliance between group therapist and patient, allows the therapist to observe the patient's reactions in the structured interpersonal setting of the interview, and reduces the number of later dropouts due to unrealistic expectations (Kanas 1995; MacKenzie 1990). The therapist assesses that the patient has an appropriate diagnosis and can tolerate sitting in the group for the entire session. If accepted, the patient is informed that this is a discussion-oriented therapy group that is designed to meet the needs of people like him- or herself who have had a nervous breakdown. The goals of the group and the types of topics discussed are summarized. The therapist informs the new patient that he or she will be expected to be on time for the sessions, to attend regularly, and to participate as much as possible. The value of learning from the other patients rather than from the therapists should be emphasized. Finally, the therapist explains that safety is paramount in the group, and for this reason none of the members are allowed to be verbally or physically abusive or threatening. As with any other patients, schizophrenic patients need to be fully informed about the nature of their treatment and to be given every opportunity to ask for clarification and to agree to participate. Because the new referral might be disorganized when initially seen by one of the therapists, much of this orienting information is repeated by the group leaders and the continuing patients at the time of the new participant's first session.

Concurrent Group and Individual Therapy

Most schizophrenic patients are seen individually for counseling and medication management, but, as has been discussed in Chapter 1, many of these patients benefit from additional psychosocial treatment as well. As has been considered, group therapy is one form of psychosocial treatment that is very valuable, but individual approaches also may be useful. Traditionally, individual therapy with psychotic patients is discussion oriented, supportive rather than uncovering, and focused on practical solutions to current problems.

In addition to this supportive therapy, a number of other individual approaches have been developed for schizophrenic patients. Many of these approaches use techniques that are similar to those described earlier in this chapter for groups of schizophrenic patients. Corrigan and Storzbach (1993) discussed three types of interventions that are based on 1) operant conditioning and reinforcement strategies, 2) training in coping skills, and 3) collaborative discussions with patients. The first type of intervention is useful when symptoms are sufficiently disruptive or bizarre to alienate other people. The second type is of value when symptoms are internally distressing to the patient. The third type is appropriate for delusions that are preventing the patient from functioning but are not internally perceived as being problematic. Breier and Strauss (1983) view the control of psychosis as being a three-phase process: self-monitoring (i.e., becoming aware of the existence of psychotic behavior), self-evaluation (i.e., recognizing the implications of these behaviors as signals of a disorder), and self-control (i.e., being able to regulate the frequency or intensity of psychotic symptoms). Patients can be taught control strategies, which Breier and Strauss view as clustering in three common areas: self-instruction, reduced involvement in activities, and increased involvement in activities. Falloon and Talbot (1981) studied 40 chronic schizophrenic outpatients and found that nearly half or more reported the following coping mechanisms to be useful in controlling their auditory hallucinations: changing their posture, engaging in some specific task or activity, initiating interpersonal contact, taking additional medications or drugs (e.g., alcohol), reducing or increasing physiological arousal (e.g., relaxing, listening to music), and cognitively altering their attention to the voices (e.g., thinking of other things). In a study of 86 schizophrenic patients, Cohen and Berk (1985) found that using self-suggestion to overpower unwanted thoughts, engaging in isolated diversions such as watching television or listening to the radio, and existentially accepting and learning to live with their symptoms were common strategies of coping, although 13% of the patients helplessly declared that they tried to gain mastery over their symptoms but failed.

Some authors have focused on specific approaches to reduce psychotic symptoms. These include humming or opening the mouth to stop the subvocal speech that is assumed to relate to auditory hallucinations (Bick and Kinsbourne 1987; Green and Kinsbourne 1990), altering auditory stimulation through ear plugs or varying amounts of noise to compensate for the interhemispheric defects and information-processing problems that are hypothesized to lead to psychotic experiences in schizophrenic patients (Chiu et al. 1988; Green and Kotenko 1980; Margo et al. 1981; Slade 1974), and cognitive-behavioral techniques that train schizophrenic patients to deal with their symptoms (Eckman et al. 1992; Meichenbaum and Cameron 1973). These specialized approaches deal with individual patients and tend to use a behavioral or educational format in helping schizophrenic patients cope with their psychotic experiences. Although none has proven to be successful for all patients under all conditions (Dobson et al. 1995; Galin et al. 1990; Geczy and Sultenfuss 1995), they represent interesting alternatives to traditional individual supportive therapy and deserve to be studied more in the future.

Research reviews that compare group with individual therapy show both approaches to be about equally effective, with a nod being given to group therapy on the basis of robustness of findings and greater treatment efficiency (Kanas 1986; MacKenzie 1990, 1994; Tillitski 1990; Toseland and Siporin 1986). For example, in a review of 32 studies that compared individual with group treatments, Toseland and Siporin (1986) found no difference between the two modalities in 24 studies, but in the remaining 8 studies, group treatment was significantly more effective. They also concluded that groups were more efficient than individual treatment in 10 of 12 studies that made this comparison, and there were fewer dropouts in groups.

Sometimes it is useful to consider using both approaches concurrently, and the pros and cons of doing this for a given patient need to be evaluated carefully (Kanas 1995; Toseland and Siporin 1986; van Montfoort and Thelosen 1994). Adding group therapy for patients in individual therapy is useful for those who cannot accept feedback from the therapists but who can accept reality-oriented advice from others who have similar problems. In addition, some schizophrenic patients are more stressed in the one-to-one situation than in a setting where others can be on the "hot seat" for some of the time. The group also provides an interpersonal laboratory where patients can practice interacting with others in a safe, controlled environment, and this is beneficial for patients who are withdrawn or who have odd ways of relating that can be examined in the here and now. Finally, blockages and resistances in individual therapy can sometimes be better exposed in the group environment, especially for patients who feel supported and are able to identify with other members of the group.

Adding individual therapy for patients in group therapy is useful for patients who need more attention due to a crisis or who suffer from complicated or sensitive problems that require a more intensive approach. Other patients find it hard to open up in a group, and the reasons for this can be explored in the individual setting. Some patients become more confused or anxious by the multiple inputs that result from the group environment, and for them individual therapy may be the only nonmedication treatment they receive until they are stabilized. Because of the attention received in the one-to-one setting, individual therapy might be considered by some patients to be better or more special, and when this becomes an issue in a group, a frank discussion of the pros and cons of these two valuable treatment approaches needs to be undertaken.

The term *combined therapy* refers to situations where the same therapist participates in both group and individual therapy, whereas the term *conjoint therapy* refers to the use of different therapists in each modality. Most therapists prefer the combined approach, because patients can be managed without the need for time-consuming communication between two or more individuals and because the splitting of different therapists into good and bad objects can be minimized. Some patients who do not have individual access to a therapist may resent other group members who do, although this competitive issue can usually be dealt with in the group. Conjoint therapy can be useful where it is necessary to diminish the intensity of the one-to-one transference or where a therapist is not well trained in both individual and group modalities. Whichever concurrent approach is used, however, individual and group therapy can complement each other when the treatment goals are specified and when the boundary between these two treatment activities is clear.

References

Bick PA, Kinsbourne M: Auditory hallucinations and subvocal speech in schizophrenic patients. Am J Psychiatry 144:222–225, 1987

Breier A, Strauss JS: Self-control in psychotic disorders. Arch Gen Psychiatry 40:1141–1145, 1983

Chiu LPW, Putkonen AR, Rimon R: Control of auditory and visual hallucinations using two behavioural techniques: a case report. Psychiatria Fennica 19:75–85, 1988

Cohen CI, Berk LA: Personal coping styles of schizophrenic outpatients. Hosp Community Psychiatry 36:407–410, 1985

Corrigan PW, Storzbach DM: Behavioral interventions for alleviating psychotic symptoms. Hosp Community Psychiatry 44:341–347, 1993

Dobson DJG, McDougall G, Busheikin J, et al: Effects of social skills training and social milieu treatment on symptoms of schizophrenia. Psychiatric Services 46:376–380, 1995

Douglas MS, Mueser KT: Teaching conflict resolution skills to the chronically ill. Behav Modif 14:519–547, 1990

Drake RE, Sederer LI: The adverse effects of intensive treatment of chronic schizophrenia. Compr Psychiatry 27:313–326, 1986

Eckman TA, Wirshing WC, Marder SR, et al: Techniques for training schizophrenic patients in illness self-management: a controlled trial. Am J Psychiatry 149:1549–1555, 1992

Falloon IRH, Talbot RE: Persistent auditory hallucinations: coping mechanisms and implications for management. Psychol Med 11:329–339, 1981

Galin D, Rodgers V, Merrin EL: Story recall under monaural and binaural conditions in psychiatric patients. Biol Psychiatry 28:794–808, 1990

Geczy B, Sultenfuss J: Group psychotherapy on state hospital admission wards. Int J Group Psychother 45:1–15, 1995

Green MF, Kinsbourne M: Subvocal activity and auditory hallucinations: clues for behavioral treatments? Schizophr Bull 16:617–625, 1990

Green P, Kotenko V: Superior speech comprehension in schizophrenics under monaural versus binaural listening conditions. J Abnorm Psychol 89:399–408, 1980

Hierholzer RW, Liberman RP: Successful living: a social skills and problem-solving group for the chronic mentally ill. Hosp Community Psychiatry 37:913–918, 1986

Kanas N: Group therapy with schizophrenics: a review of controlled studies. Int J Group Psychother 36:339–351, 1986

Kanas N: Group therapy with schizophrenic patients: a short-term, homogeneous approach. Int J Group Psychother 41:33–48, 1991

Kanas N: Group psychotherapy, in Review of General Psychiatry, 4th Edition. Edited by Goldmann HH. Norwalk, CT, Appleton & Lange, 1995, pp 454–460

Kanas N, Barr MA: Short-term homogeneous group therapy for schizophrenic inpatients: a questionnaire evaluation. Group 6:32–38, 1982

Kanas N, Barr MA: Self-control of psychotic productions in schizophrenics. Arch Gen Psychiatry 41:919–920, 1984

Kanas N, Smith AJ: Schizophrenic group process: a comparison and replication using the HIM-G. Group 14:246–252, 1990

Kanas N, Rogers M, Kreth E, et al: The effectiveness of group psychotherapy during the first three weeks of hospitalization: a controlled study. J Nerv Ment Dis 168:487–492, 1980

Kibel HD: The therapeutic use of splitting: the role of the mother-group in therapeutic differentiation and practicing, in Psychoanalytic Group Theory and Therapy. Edited by Tuttman S. Madison, CT, International Universities Press, 1991, pp 113–132

MacDonald WS, Blochberger CW, Maynard HM: Group therapy: a comparison of patient-led and staff-led groups on an open hospital ward. Psychiatr Q 38 (suppl):290–303, 1964

MacKenzie KR: Introduction to Time-Limited Group Psychotherapy. Washington, DC, American Psychiatric Press, 1990

MacKenzie KR: Where is here and when is now? the adaptational challenge of mental health reform for group psychotherapy. Int J Group Psychother 44:407–428, 1994

Margo A, Hemsley DR, Slade PD: The effects of varying auditory input on schizophrenic hallucinations. Br J Psychiatry 139:122–127, 1981

Meichenbaum D, Cameron R: Training schizophrenics to talk to themselves: a means of developing attentional controls. Behavior Therapy 4:515–534, 1973

Pattison EM, Brissenden E, Wohl T: Assessing special effects of inpatient group psychotherapy. Int J Group Psychother 17:283–297, 1967

Slade PD: The external control of auditory hallucinations: an information theory analysis. British Journal of Social and Clinical Psychology 13:73–79, 1974

Strassberg DS, Roback HB, Anchor KN, et al: Self-disclosure in group therapy with schizophrenics. Arch Gen Psychiatry 32:1259–1261, 1975

Tillitski CJ: A meta-analysis of estimated effect sizes for group versus individual versus control treatments. Int J Group Psychother 40:215–224, 1990

Toseland RW, Siporin M: When to recommend group treatment: a review of the clinical and the research literature. Int J Group Psychother 36:171–201, 1986

van Montfoort R, Thelosen E: Combined individual and group-analytic psychotherapy with young psychotics. Group Analysis 27:497–503, 1994

Weiner MF: Outcome of psychoanalytically oriented group psychotherapy. Group 8:3–12, 1984

Yalom ID: Inpatient Group Psychotherapy. New York, Basic Books, 1983

Clinical Issues: Group Process

Group process relates to the characteristics, norms, and climate of a group. It defines what is going on during a session and changes in what is going on from session to session. It includes such concepts as group dynamics, developmental stages, and therapeutic factors. Because a group's internal environment is affected not only by the specific problems of its members but also by their general outlook on life as determined by their social values, it is useful to compare a specific treatment approach across societies to look for culture-bound characteristics. Once a group's process is characterized, it can more easily be taught to others. These process issues are examined in this chapter with reference to the integrative therapy group model for schizophrenic patients, along with a consideration of the value and cost-effectiveness of this approach.

Group Dynamics

When people interact in discrete groups for any purpose, forces are set in motion that are a feature of collective human behavior. These forces are more than the simple sum of all the interactions that occur, yet they profoundly affect each member. An example is the conversion of a law-abiding person into an irrational violent criminal as a result of mob rule. The way in which these collective forces operate is the essence of group dynamics.

It is important for a therapist to be sensitive to a group's dynamics for several reasons. First, some environments are more conducive to helpful change than others, and the leader's job is to try to enhance the therapeutic potential of the group as much as possible. Second, when irrational forces threaten to retard progress or even harm a group member psychologically, the therapists can intervene with specific techniques to correct the problem and protect patient safety. Third, leaders can make observational or interpretive comments at one of three levels: to an individual patient, to two patients who are interacting inappropriately, or to the whole group (Agazarian 1983). Thus, they must continually be aware of the relative influences of group dynamics as well as intrapsychic and interpersonal dynamics in a given situation to decide at which level to intervene.

As a rule of thumb, interventions are made at the individual level when one person is having a problem; they are made at the interpersonal (dyadic) level when two people are reacting maladaptively; and they are made at the group level when three or more people seem to be affected in a similar manner. For example, if a person is hearing voices, he or she becomes the focus of the intervention. If two people are not listening to one another about a distorted belief, their inability to communicate becomes the issue. If three or more people refuse to talk about their suspicious thoughts, their general resistance or distrust becomes a possible topic for the whole group to consider.

Yalom (1975) suggested that patients learn more by talking about current issues involving each other during the sessions (the here and now) than by talking about past issues involving other people outside of the group (the there and then). The here and now has an immediacy that can be very powerful, especially when a particular symptom or interpersonal problem can be observed directly by all the group members. A here-and-now focus also is a window into the group's dynamics, because it is sensitive to the current psychological state of the members. This allows the leaders to make comments on the group process quickly, naturally, and in a way that can be appreciated by the patients.

In the integrative group approach, the leaders try to keep the focus on the here and now by encouraging the members to look at and to speak with each other about the symptoms or interpersonal problems that they are having at the present time, either during the sessions or currently on the ward or at home. If patients persist in talking about the past, the leaders may need to make a group-level intervention and point out that the members will get more out of the sessions by discussing current issues.

The therapists actively encourage discussions that are inter-active and that deal with topics that are congruent with the needs of schizophrenic patients. When they perceive the group doing this naturally and spontaneously, the leaders are silent. When they perceive that the group is becoming disorganized or quiet, they intervene to provide structure and to focus the members on a relevant topic area. When tension begins to rise in the group (e.g., members become loose or agitated or want to leave the room) or when anger or physical confrontation threatens to erupt, the leaders change the subject or comment that the group is feeling unsafe and suggest a break in the discussion.

Process studies conducted by me and my colleagues have shed some light on the environment of the groups, and these are reviewed in Chapter 7. Briefly, the groups are cohesive and dem-onstrate low levels of avoidance, conflict, and anxiety. The pa-tients are able to be confronted about significant aspects of their problems, and they exhibit little resistance. The therapists are ac-tive and define the unique parameters of the groups. The topics discussed are congruent with the group goals and generally con-sist of issues related to interacting better with others and to coping with psychotic experiences. Overall, the group climate is interac-tive, open, and safe.

Group Developmental Stages

Any living system, from the simple cell to a complex unit of gov-ernment, changes and develops over time. The same is true for therapy groups. If the group is open, significant change factors include the entry of a new patient or the departure of a patient who has completed treatment. A new group results whenever the membership changes, and the group dynamics will shift with the new cast of characters. Some regression may occur as new people become integrated and as departing people take with them a bit of the culture and the stability of the group. Thus, the process in open groups is characterized by a movement to a certain mode of functioning, alternating with a retreat to a previous mode when-ever the composition of the membership changes.

In closed groups, where the membership is relatively constant, a sequence of stages in the group process can be observed, especially in long-term settings. This sequence is more linear than is the case for open groups, and progress from one stage to another is dependent on the successful resolution of issues involving the previous stage. If this resolution is unsuccessful, groups may become blocked and fail to develop further. It is widely assumed that all closed therapy groups go through the same sequence of stages, although the length of time for each may vary from one group to another.

Most conceptual schemes address similar process issues, although the number of stages varies from three (Yalom 1975) to nine (Beck 1981). Furthermore, they have dealt almost exclusively with closed groups involving nonpsychotic patients. The groups initially are characterized by hesitant participation, the establishment of normative behavior, and the development of a cohesive environment. The members are dependent on the leader for guidance and structure. This is followed by a stage where the members begin aggressively to differentiate themselves from each other and to establish a hierarchy. Relationships are conflicted, the therapist is rebelled against, and dropouts are most likely to occur. As the members resolve their issues around differentiation, the group becomes cohesive and trusting once again, and the therapist is reintegrated as a helpful guide rather than as someone to be dependent on or as someone to fight against. Productive psychological work now can take place. The members become more intimate and open, and they view each other as unique individuals with something to offer. Interdependence grows as the members give to as well as take from the group. Learning begins to generalize to situations on the outside. Finally, the members are ready to fly on their own, and termination takes place.

Because some of our research has used the short form of a process instrument called the Group Climate Questionnaire (GCQ-S), which was developed by MacKenzie (1983, 1990), and because the GCQ-S can be used to measure stage development over time in closed therapy groups, I briefly describe this system here. The GCQ-S consists of 12 statements describing group process that can be rated on 7-point Likert scales by therapists or patients after each session. From these ratings, three dimensions of the group's climate can be constructed: engaged (an indicator of group cohesion), avoiding (an indicator of reluctance to face problems), and conflict (an indicator of interpersonal friction). MacKenzie (1990) and MacKenzie and Livesley (1983) described six stages of group development that can be defined in terms of the GCQ-S system: engagement, differentiation, individuation, intimacy, mutuality, and termination. Table 6–1 lists these stages, along with the characteristic patterns of each that can be expected on the engaged, avoiding, and conflict dimensions.

In closed integrative groups, I have been impressed that the members seem to relate better and to open up more as time goes on. Rarely is there conflict and anxiety. These clinical observations are supported by some of the GCQ-S findings, which show the absence of a sequence of discrete stages and a tendency toward a gradual increase in cohesion and a decrease in avoidance and conflict during the first 6 months of the groups' existence (Kanas et al. 1984, 1989a). These results are echoed in a process study of the second 15 months of a schizophrenic group by Isbell et al. (1992), where it was concluded that the group functioned at a high and increasing level of cohesion without evidence of discrete stages over time using the Group Environment Scale.

It is possible that groups involving schizophrenic patients do not have the same developmental sequence as groups of nonpsychotic patients due to the inability of schizophrenic patients to tolerate anxiety and strong affect. Groups involving neurotic and characterological patients must go through a stage of differentia-

Table 6–1.   Group developmental stages and the short form of the Group Climate Questionnaire

Stage	Dimension scores		
	Engaged	**Avoiding**	**Conflict**
1. Engagement	High	Low	Low
2. Differentiation	Low	High	High
3. Individuation	High	Low	Low
4. Intimacy	High	High	Low
5. Mutuality	High	Low	High
6. Termination	No characteristic pattern reported		

tion and conflict before they can progress to later stages of intimacy and mutuality. Groups of schizophrenic patients may become blocked from moving into these later stages due to the poor tolerance of these patients for the stresses that occur in the stage of differentiation. Alternatively, perhaps the focus on safety and support holds the patients back at an early stage of group development by not allowing them to experience and deal with strong affect and conflict during the sessions. This artifact of technique would then apply more to the integrative model than to other approaches. However, others also have found schizophrenic patients to be intolerant of anxiety and strong negative emotions (Drake and Sederer 1986; Geczy and Sultenfuss 1995; Kanas et al. 1980; MacDonald et al. 1964; Pattison et al. 1967; Strassberg et al. 1975; Weiner 1984).

Whatever the reasons for the GCQ-S findings, however, a group environment where schizophrenic patients become more trusting and open with one another as time goes on is a positive thing. The patients are not expected to gain developmental insight or to work through early anxiety-producing traumatic conflicts. Rather, they are being asked to share strategies of coping with symptoms and to learn ways of relating better with other people. With these goals in mind, perhaps a pattern of increasing cohesion and decreasing avoidance and conflict is an appropriate way for a therapy group composed of schizophrenic patients to develop over time, at least for the first 6 months or so of its existence.

Therapeutic Factors

One important aspect of group process pertains to the factors that contribute to the improvement in a patient's condition. MacKenzie (1990) described four kinds: supportive factors, self-revelation factors, learning from others factors, and psychological work factors. Based on a review of the literature, Bloch et al. (1981) isolated 10 specific therapeutic factors that apply to therapy groups: acceptance (cohesiveness), altruism, catharsis, existential factors, guidance, insight, instillation of hope, interaction, self-disclosure, and vicarious learning.

Yalom (1975) described a method of studying these therapeutic qualities of a group, which he called curative factors. At the time of discharge, patients are given 60 statements describing

12 potentially useful attributes of their group experience, and they rate these statements in terms of helpfulness. The ranking of the statements then is used to create a similar ranking of the 12 curative factors. These factors are altruism (helping others); catharsis (expressing held-in feelings); existential factors (learning to cope with the futility of life); family reenactment (reliving family issues); group cohesiveness (feeling a part of the group); guidance (receiving advice); identification (imitating qualities of others); insight or self-understanding (becoming aware of unconscious motivations and conflicts); instillation of hope (feeling optimistic by watching others improve); interpersonal learning, input (receiving feedback on interpersonal behavior); interpersonal learning, output (learning how to deal with other people); and universality (feeling less isolated from others).

This method of ranking a group's curative factors based on patient evaluation has been used in a number of studies. Two of these are summarized in Table 6–2. As shown in the table, Yalom's (1975) psychiatric outpatients most valued their long-term closed group for giving them feedback on interpersonal behavior, allowing them an opportunity to ventilate their feelings, giving them

Table 6–2.   Group therapy curative factors

Rank	Psychiatric outpatients (Yalom 1975)	Psychiatric inpatients (Maxmen 1973)
1	Interpersonal input	Instillation of hope
2	Catharsis	Group cohesiveness
3	Group cohesiveness	Altruism
4	Insight	Universality
5	Interpersonal output	Interpersonal input
6	Existential factors	Existential factors
7	Universality	Interpersonal output
8	Instillation of hope	Catharsis
9	Altruism	Insight
10	Family reenactment	Guidance
11	Guidance	Family reenactment
12	Identification	Identification

a sense of acceptance by other people, and helping them become aware of unconscious motivations and conflicts. In contrast, in a study of 100 psychiatric inpatients, Maxmen (1973) found a different ranking. His patients most valued their short-term open group for making them optimistic by watching others improve, giving them a sense of acceptance, improving their self-esteem by seeing they could help others, and allowing them to feel less isolated. As may be inferred from Table 6–2, the qualities deemed helpful in a therapy group can vary according to several factors, such as the type of patients in the group, the setting, and the number of sessions.

My colleagues and I have not used Yalom's (1975) 60-statement method in evaluating the integrative groups because it does not place emphasis on the needs of psychotic patients. However, we have constructed a discharge questionnaire that includes 13 therapeutic factor statements, some similar to Yalom's and some developed by us specifically for schizophrenic patients. We used this questionnaire to study both an inpatient group (Kanas and Barr 1982) and an outpatient group (Kanas et al. 1988). The rankings are shown in Table 6–3.

The two rankings correlated significantly with each other, suggesting that the patients found similar characteristics helpful in both settings. The groups were valued more as a place to learn ways of interacting with others, to test reality and cope with psychotic experiences, and to express feelings than as a place to gain insight and to receive guidance concerning their illness, medications, and economic situation. Specific statements that addressed Yalom's (1975) constructs of universality and altruism were ranked second and fourth, respectively, in the inpatient group, and they tied for fourth in the outpatient group. In both settings, a statement related to gaining insight and three statements related to receiving advice were rated eighth or lower. Both rankings of therapeutic factors seemed to be conceptually more similar to Maxmen's (1973) ranking than to Yalom's, which makes sense because Maxmen's inpatient group included schizophrenic patients and other acutely disturbed patients, whereas Yalom's group was composed of higher-functioning patients. In addition, the number of sessions averaged by Maxmen's patients (9 sessions) was more similar to our inpatient and outpatient group averages (9 and 12 sessions, respectively) than Yalom's average of approximately 64 sessions. Thus, the patients in the three short-term samples had a similar amount of group experience, and this differed greatly from Yalom's long-term sample.

Other features of the integrative approach provide therapeu-

Table 6–3. Schizophrenic group therapeutic factors questionnaire

Statement	Inpatient rank (Kanas and Barr 1982)	Outpatient rank (Kanas et al. 1988)
The group allowed me a place to express my emotions.	1	7
The group showed me that I am not the only one with problems.	2	4
The group helped me become less suspicious of others.	3	1
The group showed me that I can help other people.	4	4
The group taught me how to relate better with people.	5	2
The group helped me decide the difference between reality and my imagination.	6	2
The group helped me cope better with my voices and/or visions.	7	8
The group helped me feel hopeful about my future.	7	6
The group gave me insight into the causes of my problems.	9	8
The group gave me useful advice about the nature of my illness.	10	8
The group gave me useful advice about medications.	10	8
The group helped me learn to control some of my emotions.	12	12
The group gave me useful advice about jobs, finances, or places to stay.	13	12

tic benefit. In both inpatient and outpatient settings, the groups seem to function at a high level of work, with the members being confronted about significant aspects of their problems in a safe and open environment that shows little group resistance. The therapists are active in keeping the group on task, and they are the major influences in determining the unique qualities of the groups (Kanas and Smith 1990; Kanas et al. 1985). Cohesion may be similar to or even higher than in other therapy groups, and avoidance, conflict, and anxiety are low (N. Kanas, unpublished study, August 1994 [see Chapter 7]; Kanas et al. 1989a). Important discussion topics deal with improving interactions with others and coping with schizophrenic symptoms, and topics related to receiving advice about the nature of the illness, medications, and economic situation are relatively uncommon (N. Kanas, unpublished study, August 1994 [see Chapter 7]; Kanas and Barr 1986; Kanas et al. 1988, 1989a). Most of these process characteristics are congruent with the needs of schizophrenic patients and the goals of the group approach.

Finally, the emphasis on patient-to-patient interactions during the sessions is therapeutic in two ways. First, the members learn ways of dealing with their problems through topics discussed with others who have "been there." In addition to the more common coping strategies that one might expect, novel solutions are offered as well. For example, some of the patients report that their auditory hallucinations disappear or at least decrease in intensity when they go into an isolated area and scream at their voices to go away. Second, in the process of sharing ideas, the group members are interacting, and they are encouraged to look at and to direct their comments to each other. Thus, they are practicing important interpersonal skills in the here and now that can be generalized to interactions that occur outside of the group.

Cultural Perspectives

In the United States, groups using the integrative model have been conducted in general psychiatric settings and in special culture-sensitive units consisting of African Americans and of Asian immigrants and Asian Americans. These groups also have been started on inpatient psychiatric units in Russia (Kanas 1991a) and in England (see Chapter 7), and articles describing this model have been translated into Japanese (Kanas 1992a, 1992b). Clinical and empirical findings have supported the value of the approach in these varied settings, and local staff and trainees have been able to conceptualize and apply the techniques in a relatively brief period of time. Schizophrenic patients suffer from similar symptoms and relationship problems all over the world, and a treatment strategy that addresses these needs is bound to be relevant internationally. However, there are some culture-specific issues that clinicians need to be aware of, and it is to these that I now turn. Keep in mind that any conclusions that result are limited to the settings described earlier.

At one busy public sector general hospital located in a large city, culture-sensitive units were set up that were oriented around the special needs of patients from large minority groups that lived in the city. One such unit had a special focus on problems affecting African American patients. Most of the staff and patients were black, and the program was sensitive to issues involving discrimination and African American culture. I was the supervisor for a schizophrenic group in this program, and the therapists included a white social worker and several black nurses. Although the group generally was able to keep to its stated goals, it sometimes was diverted from these goals by social issues that keenly interested the patients.

For example,

One group session began with a discussion of suspicious thoughts, and this progressed to a consideration of how to test the reality of a suspicion that may or may not be true. Alvin, an angry paranoid schizophrenic patient, blurted out that he could not trust any white people, and he alluded to a white conspiracy against all blacks that permeated the country. When one of the therapists (a black nurse) challenged the universality of this assertion, other patients started to agree with Alvin, and the discussion began to focus on social issues involving discrimination. The group leaders pointed out that there were other times in the program where such topics could be addressed, and they tried to reframe the discussion in terms of reality testing and patient symptomatology. The group members wanted no part of this, however, and they continued to focus on their feelings about discrimination until the session ended.

In this group, emotional social issues that affected these patients as African Americans became fused with issues that pertained to their specific illness (e.g., psychotic symptomatology), despite the fact that the former were addressed elsewhere in the program. In some sessions, the patients needed to ventilate their feelings about discrimination for awhile before they could hear the therapists' comments about testing reality and dealing with their symptoms. As long as the patients were interacting and receiving support from each other, they at least were able to practice improving their social skills in the here and now of the sessions.

On a similar unit for Asian immigrants and Asian Americans, a group was started for schizophrenic patients. Because several cultural groups were represented, it was decided to conduct the sessions in English. This eliminated a few recent immigrants who were fluent only in their native language. However, other patients, even some who spoke English, reported a fear of losing "face" by being in the group and admitting to their problems in front of others, and they refused to attend. This created a danger that the group would not have enough members to support the sessions. We dealt with this issue by admitting non-Asian schizophrenic patients to the group who were from an adjoining ward. The resulting cultural heterogeneity did not present any problems because the patients were diagnostically homogeneous, and we were able to sustain enough of a critical mass to continue with the sessions. Unfortunately, we were not able to serve those patients who did not attend the group due to language and "face" issues. Perhaps if we had had enough patients (and therapists) who were fluent in the same non-English language to start a second group, the concerns about saving face might have been successfully addressed.

The issue of the members' reluctance to speak in a therapy group may reflect more on the therapists than on the patients. This can be due to inexperience and poor technique, but it also can be due to the political situation in a country and the therapists' perceptions of how their patients are reacting to it.

For example,

I supervised an inpatient group located on the female wing of a large psychiatric teaching hospital in Russia, which at the time was still the Soviet Union. Due to glasnost, Soviet society was becoming more open, and there was a great deal of interest in new psychotherapeutic approaches at the hospital. The group was conducted in the Russian language and was composed of four female schizophrenic patients and two therapists (a female clinical psychologist and a male psychiatric resident). Along with a translator, I observed the sessions from the corner of the room outside of the group circle. During the first session, I noted that the therapists seemed quite deferential to the patients. They would hesitate to probe into personal matters, would not follow up clues that the patients might be experiencing psychotic symptoms, and would even ask the patients' permission to inquire about their feelings. The patients generally were quiet, did not interact much with each other, and minimally responded to the therapists' questions. After the session, I suggested to the therapists that they should be more confrontive and ask the patients directly if they heard voices, felt suspicious, experienced confused thoughts, or had problems relating with others. Furthermore, I described some techniques that they could use to get the patients to interact more with each other. The therapists were reluctant to do this, saying that Soviet people had learned to become more private and guarded than their American counterparts, and that the doctor-patient relationship was more formal in the Soviet Union than in the United States. Nevertheless, I persisted with my advice.

The next session began in much the same manner as the previous one. However, midway through, the psychologist asked one of the patients if she heard voices. The patient said yes and added that it was hard for her to say this in front of other people. When the therapist asked the other patients to comment, they were very supportive and began describing their own psychotic experiences. After the session, the therapists expressed surprise at how much the patients revealed and how readily they responded to this gentle confrontation. They were much more direct and active in subsequent sessions, and the patients responded accordingly.

The reluctance of the therapists to confront the patients may have been due to their inexperience in leading this new group. However, it also reflected an attitude that was based on past experience with patients who had been brought up in a closed society. This might have been compounded by the fact that the interpreter and I were in the room. However, when their symptoms were addressed, the patients were open to talking about them, and the group began to behave like its counterparts in the United States and elsewhere. The symptomatic and relationship needs of schizophrenic patients transcend national boundaries, and they often respond to appropriate treatments despite political and cultural restrictions.

Cultural issues also seemed to have been transcended in an inpatient schizophrenic group that was conducted at a general hospital in a large city in England. Although most of the patients were British subjects, some were born in different countries, and they were quite diverse demographically. For example, of the 20 patients who participated in the first 10 sessions of the group's existence, 12 were male; there were 10 blacks, 8 whites, and 2 Asians. In addition, the patients in the group were from two separate units, each with its own staff and programs. Despite this diversity, the group scored significantly higher than groups in the United States on a measure of cohesion, and 77% of the discussion topics that were recorded dealt with issues that were related to coping with psychotic experiences and to interacting better with others. Although a number of factors may have accounted for these findings (see Chapter 7), they suggest that diverse groups of schizophrenic patients are able to bond together around their common illness and to focus on topics relevant to the group goals.

Training and Supervision

The treatment model presented in this book has been taught to a number of mental health staff and trainees. There is evidence that the group environment that results from this training is the same, even though the therapists and patients differ and even though the setting is inpatient or outpatient (Kanas and Smith 1990). Clinically, the model has been exported successfully to countries other than the United States. Using a combination of training and supervision, I have found that the basic techniques usually can be taught within 3 months.

The training model that I like to use for ongoing inpatient groups begins with the trainees attending lectures on the group, reading some of the relevant clinical and empirical papers, and viewing videotapes of previous group sessions. For those trainees who are strong advocates of the medical model, it is useful to expose them to the literature supporting the value of psychosocial interventions in treating schizophrenic patients (Africa and Schwartz 1992; Breier and Strauss 1983; Cohen and Berk 1985; Corrigan and Storzbach 1993; Dobson et al. 1995; Engel 1980; Falloon and Talbot 1981; Kanas and Barr 1984; Kaplan and Sadock 1989). After some of the integrative group techniques are discussed with a supervisor, the trainees watch experienced therapists conducting a group through a one-way mirror or seated in the room outside of the group circle.

The one-way mirror scenario has the advantage of allowing the trainees (as well as interested staff) to watch and discuss the group process in real time with the supervisor. It is important for all observers to introduce themselves to the patients prior to the beginning of the session, for confidentiality reasons. In addition, the patients are less suspicious and react more naturally in the group if they know who is behind the mirror. Anyone coming late who has not been introduced will not be allowed to observe. Sometimes when a number of people are observing, the group discussion begins to focus on issues of trust in an obvious reference to the people behind the mirror. The therapists need to be sensitive to this and to raise the here-and-now issue of being observed as a topic for discussion. If the patients persist in being suspicious, I sometimes turn on the light in the observing room, which allows them to see who is watching through the mirror (the mirror "reverses" itself when the observing room is brighter than the treatment room).

When the session ends and the patients leave, all of the observers join the two therapists for a 10- to 15-minute rehash of what transpired. After a few sessions, one of the trainees usually feels ready to begin, and he or she joins an experienced leader as a co-therapist. Again, the observers and therapists conduct a rehash after the session ends. This goes on until each new leader has functioned as a co-therapist with an experienced staff member for several sessions, at which point the trainees may be allowed to work with each other.

The supervisor must be respectful of the therapists and must be sensitive to the fact that they are allowing their work to be observed in front of trainees and other staff. By addressing comments to the group process and to technical issues, learning can occur in a spirit of collegiality. This group supervision is not the place to comment on an individual's performance; private sessions between supervisor and trainee should be scheduled for this purpose.

In closed outpatient groups, the same individuals may function as co-therapists throughout the life of the group. Consequently, if the trainee is quite new to group therapy, he or she needs to be paired with a more experienced co-therapist. In cases where the trainees have done similar groups before (e.g., an inpatient schizophrenic group), they can lead the group together. Either way, it is best if the supervisor observes their work directly through a one-way mirror or seated in the room outside of the group circle. Because outpatient groups usually meet less frequently but for a longer period of time than inpatient groups, the postsession rehash might last for 30 or more minutes.

In some outpatient training programs, a new trainee periodically replaces another due to a change in rotation. Thus, in a long-term group, changes in leadership may be expected to occur every 6–12 months. Schizophrenic patients may respond to such disruptions with disappointment, anger, or suspicion, and their feelings about this change need to be addressed. I usually begin reminding the group members of this occurrence at least a month before the event to allow plenty of time to discuss it. Similarly, departing trainees have feelings about leaving, and this becomes an issue for consideration during the rehash or in a private supervisory session. In inpatient settings, the frequent patient turnover makes therapist departures less of an issue, and goodbyes usually can be made during the last session.

At times, I have co-led the group with a trainee and then been the supervisor during the rehash. A common occurrence is for the trainee to defer to me (or any other experienced co-therapist) during the early sessions, and this becomes a major supervisory issue. At some point, the trainees begin to find themselves thinking of things to say just before I say them in the group. I point out that this usually means they are understanding the treatment model and are becoming sensitized to the group process and are reacting to it at about the same time as I am. At this point, most trainees become more active and are willing to take chances by offering their interventions.

There are other issues that commonly come up in supervision. Due to a lack of self-confidence or a preconceived notion of how to lead therapy groups, many trainees are not prepared to be as active in structuring the group discussions as they sometimes need to be. They let the patients drift off the topic or use up group time discussing an issue that is not relevant to the group goals. I point out that time management is important in these groups and that the sequence of identification then generalization then coping ideally will occur in every session (see Chapter 5). I also tell the trainees that the patients should be discussing coping strategies by the last half or third of the session. Other trainees are too active, sometimes interrupting patients who are talking with each other and bringing the focus of the group members' attention onto themselves. I stress the therapeutic value of patient-to-patient interactions, and we discuss ways to encourage this. Finally, some trainees make interventions that are too wordy or abstract. I point out that psychotic patients often are confused and disorganized and that their mental state may change from time to time due to stress and to medication side effects. Consequently, group therapists need to be mindful of making short, concrete, and clear comments that may need to be repeated from time to time to be fully understood and processed by the patients.

Value and Cost-Effectiveness of the Groups

The evidence to date supports the value of the integrative approach for patients. Both inpatients and outpatients have rated their group experience as being helpful (Kanas and Barr 1982; Kanas et al. 1988), which is consistent with clinical impressions and the feedback received from program staff. Some outpatients have experienced reductions in symptoms and social anxiety, and they have reported improvement in relating with others and in coping with psychotic experiences for up to 4 months after the group has ended (Kanas et al. 1988, 1989b). More than half of the outpatients who complete a short-term group choose to participate in a similar group experience within 2 years (Kanas 1991b; Kanas and Smith 1990). Finally, patients regularly come to the sessions. Attendance rates typically are in the 80%–90% range, and outpatient dropout rates generally are less than 20% (Kanas and Smith 1990; Kanas et al. 1984, 1989a, 1989b).

Several lines of reasoning support the cost-effectiveness of the integrative groups as well. First, group therapy in general is an efficient modality of treatment. Retrospective analysis of health insurance claims data and meta-analysis of controlled studies have converged to show that psychotherapy (including group therapy) provides a cost-offset effect in terms of reducing subsequent medical services (Mumford et al. 1984). When comparing various forms of group and individual therapy, the former modality is more cost-effective. For example, Toseland and Siporin (1986) found group treatment to be more efficient than individual treatment in 10 of 12 studies that made this comparison. Also, MacKenzie (1994) reported that the overall utilization of clinician time using group methods is less than half that using individual approaches and that the mean number of sessions for patients using group therapy is 8 visits, as compared with 20 visits using individual therapy. There is evidence that 8 therapy visits is a kind of plateau that is typical and useful for most patients. For example, in outpatient settings, nearly 85% of patients attend 8 or fewer therapy sessions, and more than half of them improve. In contrast, less than 10% of patients attend 26 or more sessions, and these account for only a quarter of the total number improved (MacKenzie 1990, 1994). Thus, the majority of patients do not require long-term therapy, and short-term treatment approaches are very cost-effective, especially those using group therapy.

A second line of reasoning that supports the cost-effectiveness of our groups relates to two observations: 1) patients who are treated in inpatient groups are more likely to participate in outpatient groups (Yalom 1983), and 2) in the aftercare setting, therapy groups for schizophrenic patients lower rehospitalization rates and decrease the time spent in the hospital during subsequent readmissions (Alden et al. 1979; Battegay and von Marschall 1978; Shattan et al. 1966). Therefore, participation in inpatient integrative groups would be expected to improve the likelihood of participation in similar outpatient groups, and this in turn should contribute to fewer hospital days in the future. In addition, because our groups focus on helping schizophrenic patients improve their interpersonal relationships and become more reality oriented, these patients are better able to cooperate with outpatient treatment staff and interact more appropriately with family, friends, board and care operators, and so on. This not only improves the quality of their lives, but it also leads to increased compliance with treatment and reduces the likelihood of rehospitalization.

Third, our integrative groups average two therapists and six to eight patients per session. This represents a staff-to-patient ratio of 1:3 or 1:4 during the 45–60 minutes that the groups meet. This is an efficient use of staff time, especially when the cotherapy team includes trainees. In addition, the per-patient time taken to chart a therapy session is relatively brief, because our therapists typically take turns writing a common "process note" that is copied and placed in each member's medical record. (For confidentiality reasons, each patient is identified by his or her initials so that a reader of patient A's records will not be able to guess the identity of patient B, and so on.)

Fourth, our group model encourages patients to learn from and to interact with others in a multiperson context, something that cannot occur in individual therapy. This provides an opportunity for them to practice new interpersonal skills and to receive valuable feedback from people who have similar problems, all in a controlled setting. Many schizophrenic patients find that this format addresses their needs, and they do not have to engage in more staff-intensive individual therapies.

Finally, recent trends in health care have mandated the use of treatment approaches that are not only helpful but are also brief. As described earlier, therapy groups of about 8 sessions in length have been found to be efficient and effective. Many of our integrative groups approach this duration, with patients typically attending an average of 9 inpatient sessions or 12 outpatient sessions in our time-limited clinic groups (Kanas 1991b). Although the argument is made that schizophrenia is a chronic mental illness that requires long-term follow-up, many of our outpatients report being able to continue gains they have made for several months after the group ends (Kanas et al. 1988, 1989b), and nearly half feel that one trial of 12 sessions is enough when they are offered another group experience 1–2 years later (Kanas 1991b; Kanas and Smith 1990). Patients who desire more treatment can join a second 12-session "repeater's" group. Whereas most schizophrenic patients need to be followed for support and medication management on a more or less continuous basis, this is not to say that all will require long-term group therapy. For those who do not, a program that offers participation in sequential, time-limited, 12-session group therapy blocks offers a more cost-effective alternative.

References

Africa B, Schwartz SR: Schizophrenic disorders, in Review of General Psychiatry, 3rd Edition. Edited by Goldman HH. Norwalk, CT, Appleton & Lange, 1992, pp 198–214

Agazarian YM: Theory of the invisible group applied to individual and group-as-a-whole interpretations. Group 7:27–37, 1983

Alden AR, Weddington WW Jr, Jacobson C, et al: Group aftercare for chronic schizophrenia. J Clin Psychiatry 40:249–252, 1979

Battegay R, von Marschall R: Results of long-term group psychotherapy with schizophrenics. Compr Psychiatry 19:349–353, 1978

Beck AP: Developmental characteristics of the system-forming process, in Living Groups: Group Psychotherapy and General System Theory. Edited by Durkin JE. New York, Brunner/Mazel, 1981, pp 316–332

Bloch S, Crouch E, Reibstein J: Therapeutic factors in group psychotherapy. Arch Gen Psychiatry 38:519–526, 1981

Breier A, Strauss JS: Self-control in psychotic disorders. Arch Gen Psychiatry 40:1141–1145, 1983

Cohen CI, Berk LA: Personal coping styles of schizophrenic outpatients. Hosp Community Psychiatry 36:407–410, 1985

Corrigan PW, Storzbach DM: Behavioral interventions for alleviating psychotic symptoms. Hosp Community Psychiatry 44:341–347, 1993

Dobson DJG, McDougall G, Busheikin J, et al: Effects of social skills training and social milieu treatment on symptoms of schizophrenia. Psychiatric Services 46:376–380, 1995

Drake RE, Sederer LI: The adverse effects of intensive treatment of chronic schizophrenia. Compr Psychiatry 27:313–326, 1986

Engel GL: The clinical application of the biopsychosocial model. Am J Psychiatry 137:535–544, 1980

Falloon IRH, Talbot RE: Persistent auditory hallucinations: coping mechanisms and implications for management. Psychol Med 11:329–339, 1981

Geczy B, Sultenfuss J: Group psychotherapy on state hospital admission wards. Int J Group Psychother 45:1–15, 1995

Isbell SE, Thorne A, Lawler MH: An exploratory study of videotapes of long-term group psychotherapy of outpatients with major and chronic mental illness. Group 16:101–111, 1992

Kanas N: Group therapy in Leningrad. Group 15:14–22, 1991a

Kanas N: Group therapy with schizophrenic patients: a short-term, homogeneous approach. Int J Group Psychother 41:33–48, 1991b

Kanas N: Group therapy with schizophrenic patients: a short-term, homogeneous approach (translated in Japanese). Journal of the Japan Association of Group Psychotherapy 8:83–92, 1992a

Kanas N: Group therapy with schizophrenics: American and Japanese perspectives (in Japanese and English). Journal of the Japan Association of Group Psychotherapy 8:100–102, 1992b

Kanas N, Barr MA: Short-term homogeneous group therapy for schizophrenic inpatients: a questionnaire evaluation. Group 6:32–38, 1982

Kanas N, Barr MA: Self-control of psychotic productions in schizophrenics. Arch Gen Psychiatry 41:919–920, 1984

Kanas N, Barr MA: Process and content in a short-term inpatient schizophrenic group. Small Group Behavior 17:355–363, 1986

Kanas N, Smith AJ: Schizophrenic group process: a comparison and replication using the HIM-G. Group 14:246–252, 1990

Kanas N, Rogers M, Kreth E, et al: The effectiveness of group psychotherapy during the first three weeks of hospitalization: a controlled study. J Nerv Ment Dis 168:487–492, 1980

Kanas N, DiLella VJ, Jones J: Process and content in an outpatient schizophrenic group. Group 8:13–20, 1984

Kanas N, Barr MA, Dossick S: The homogeneous schizophrenic inpatient group: an evaluation using the Hill Interaction Matrix. Small Group Behavior 16:397–409, 1985

Kanas N, Stewart P, Haney K: Content and outcome in a short-term therapy group for schizophrenic outpatients. Hosp Community Psychiatry 39:437–439, 1988

Kanas N, Stewart P, Deri J, et al: Group process in short-term outpatient therapy groups for schizophrenics. Group 13:67–73, 1989a

Kanas N, Deri J, Ketter T, et al: Short-term outpatient therapy groups for schizophrenics. Int J Group Psychother 39:517–522, 1989b

Kaplan HI, Sadock BJ (eds): Comprehensive Textbook of Psychiatry, 5th Edition. Baltimore, MD, Williams & Wilkins, 1989

MacDonald WS, Blochberger CW, Maynard HM: Group therapy: a comparison of patient-led and staff-led groups on an open hospital ward. Psychiatr Q 38 (suppl):290–303, 1964

MacKenzie KR: The clinical application of a group climate measure, in Advances in Group Psychotherapy: Integrating Research and Practice. Edited by Dies RR, MacKenzie KR. New York, International Universities Press, 1983, pp 159–170

MacKenzie KR: Introduction to Time-Limited Group Psychotherapy. Washington, DC, American Psychiatric Press, 1990

MacKenzie KR: Where is here and when is now?: the adaptational challenge of mental health reform for group psychotherapy. Int J Group Psychother 44:407–428, 1994

MacKenzie KR, Livesley WJ: A developmental model for brief group therapy, in Advances in Group Psychotherapy: Integrating Research and Practice. Edited by Dies RR, MacKenzie KR. New York, International Universities Press, 1983, pp 101–116

Maxmen JS: Group therapy as viewed by hospitalized patients. Arch Gen Psychiatry 28:404–408, 1973

Mumford E, Schlesinger HJ, Glass GV, et al: A new look at evidence about reduced cost of medical utilization following mental health treatment. Am J Psychiatry 141:1145–1158, 1984

Pattison EM, Brissenden E, Wohl T: Assessing special effects of inpatient group psychotherapy. Int J Group Psychother 17:283–297, 1967

Shattan SP, D'Camp L, Fujii E, et al: Group treatment of conditionally discharged patients in a mental health clinic. Am J Psychiatry 122:798–805, 1966

Strassberg DS, Roback HB, Anchor KN, et al: Self-disclosure in group therapy with schizophrenics. Arch Gen Psychiatry 32:1259–1261, 1975

Toseland RW, Siporin M: When to recommend group treatment: a review of the clinical and the research literature. Int J Group Psychother 36:171–201, 1986

Weiner MF: Outcome of psychoanalytically oriented group psychotherapy. Group 8:3–12, 1984

Yalom ID: The Theory and Practice of Group Psychotherapy, 2nd Edition. New York, Basic Books, 1975

Yalom ID: Inpatient Group Psychotherapy. New York, Basic Books, 1983

CHAPTER 7

Research Issues

*T*he integrative group therapy model described in the preceding chapters has developed from and been supported by a number of empirical studies conducted by me and my colleagues since 1975. These have included studies of outcome, process, and content (i.e., discussion topics). In this chapter, this research is reviewed in two broad categories: inpatient studies and outpatient studies. Although the highlights are presented, the interested reader is referred to the original articles for specific details.

Inpatient Studies

The first study began in 1975 on a 25-bed psychiatric clinical research unit located in a large military teaching hospital. The patients included active duty personnel, their dependents, and military retirees. We were interested in evaluating the effectiveness of group therapy for acute psychiatric inpatients. Following a 3-month pilot phase (Kanas et al. 1978), newly admitted patients who signed informed consent were randomly assigned to one of three experimental conditions: group therapy; activities-oriented task group; or control condition, where the patients were not involved with small groups. The therapy group treatment model utilized an insight-oriented, uncovering approach and included both psychotic and nonpsychotic members. At the time, this model was used on many inpatient units, and it was only after the study ended that we became fully aware of the potential dangers of an insight-oriented approach for psychotic individuals (Drake and Sederer 1986; Geczy and Sultenfuss 1995; Kanas et al. 1980; MacDonald et al. 1964; Pattison et al. 1967; Strassberg et al. 1975; Weiner 1984).

The patients participated in each condition for 1 hour three times per week (those in the control condition were given free time on the ward during this time). They were evaluated shortly after admission and after 8 experimental days (which averaged 20 days postadmission for all three conditions) by nurse evaluators who were blind to the experimental condition. A number of measures were used, including the Psychiatric Evaluation Form, the Global Assessment Scale, and a behavioral measure that quantified a patient's ward privileges (e.g., suicide precautions, restricted to ward, free to sign out for weekend passes) on a 1–9 scale. These privileges were determined by a consensus of patients and staff during community meetings. Patient medication use and individual therapy contact times also were recorded on special research forms.

A total of 86 patients completed the study (44% were psychotic, nearly all of whom were schizophrenic, and 63% were male). The results showed that the majority of patients improved, and there were no significant differences in improvement rates between patients in the three conditions (Kanas et al. 1980). As expected, there were no differences across conditions in medication use or individual therapy contact times. However, significantly more psychotic patients who were assigned to group therapy got *worse* than psychotic patients who were assigned to the other two conditions. Table 7–1 shows this in terms of the Psychiatric Evaluation Form overall severity of illness measure and the percentage of patients who dropped in ward privilege status from admission to second evaluation. There were no significant differences in decrement rate across conditions for nonpsychotic patients. We concluded that group therapy did not offer a measurable advantage over an activities group and a no-small-group control condition for acute inpatients during the first 3 weeks of hospitalization. Furthermore, it seemed that this treatment modality was harmful for schizophrenic patients, especially in our mixed psychotic/nonpsychotic groups that utilized an insight-oriented approach.

Troubled by these findings, I became interested in developing a treatment approach whereby schizophrenic patients could be treated safely and effectively in group therapy. After I took a position in 1977 with the University of California and the Department of Veterans Affairs (VA) in San Francisco, I began working with Dr. Mary Ann Barr on a clinical approach that would be useful for acutely psychotic schizophrenic inpatients. What resulted was a supportive, homogeneous model that did not utilize insight-oriented, uncovering techniques but instead focused on ways that the patients could cope with psychotic symptoms and improve their interpersonal relationships. The group that we co-led met three times per week and was open to schizophrenic patients who were admitted to a 30-bed acute-care psychiatric inpatient unit at a VA hospital. Most of the patients were male veterans, and the average length of stay on this open unit was 3 weeks, although the schizophrenic patients tended to remain about 5 weeks due to medication management and placement issues. The program emphasized a multimodal, multidisciplinary approach that included individual counseling, community meetings, occupational and recreational therapy, and psychotropic medications. After we became comfortable with our clinical model, we began to study the group empirically.

In the first study (Kanas and Barr 1982), we administered a

Table 7–1. Percentage of psychotic patients getting worse during the first 20 days of hospitalization

Condition	Increases in Psychiatric Evaluation Form overall severity of illness		Drops in ward privilege	
	Patients (%)	P^a	Patients (%)	P^a
No small group	0		20	
Therapy group	38	.03	56	.07
Activities group	17	NS	17	.03

^{a}For both measures, the differences between the no small group and the activities group conditions were nonsignificant (NS) ($P > .10$).

discharge questionnaire to 22 male schizophrenic patients who had participated in the group for an average of nine sessions. On the questionnaire, the patients were first asked to assess how helpful the group had been for them, then to rate 13 statements that described a number of factors that we thought might be therapeutic; 95% rated the group as "very" or "somewhat" helpful. Significantly more patients below the median age of 29.5 years found the group very helpful than did patients above the median age, and significantly more nonparanoid schizophrenic patients found the group very helpful than did paranoid schizophrenic patients. There were no significant differences in overall satisfaction that were related to race or number of sessions attended. In examining the ranking of therapeutic factors, the patients valued the group more as a place to express emotions, to learn ways of relating better with others, and to test reality and cope with psychotic experiences than as a place to gain insight into the causes of their problems or to receive practical advice on their illness, medications, or economic situation (see Table 6–3 in Chapter 6). Coupled with our own clinical impressions and positive feedback from the ward staff, these results suggested that we were on the right track. The patients indicated that they found the group to be helpful and valued it for dealing with issues that were related to their illness.

In a second inpatient study, we evaluated the characteristics of the group using the Hill Interaction Matrix. This well-known process measure has been used for more than 30 years and classifies therapy groups in terms of what is being discussed (content style) and the manner in which the groups help the members learn about themselves (work style). The four content style categories (topic [I], group [II], personal [III], and relationship [IV]) and the four active work style categories (conventional [B], assertive [C], speculative [D], and confrontive [E]) interact to form a 4 × 4 matrix of 16 cells that are named by their content and work components (e.g., IB, IIIE). The category and matrix scores for a group under study can then be compared with similar scores from a normative sample of 50 therapy group sessions. In addition, ratios that give important clinical information can be calculated. One of these is the Th/M ratio, which indicates that the therapists (Th) are contributing more than the patient members (M) in a particular category or matrix cell if the value is above 1.00. We used a form of the Hill Interaction Matrix called the HIM-G. This measure is composed of 72 items rated by a group observer that describe such things as the percentage of therapist time involved in either initiating or maintaining the group member interactions that are characteristic of each of the 16 cells, the percentage of patient time and the number of patients involved in the typical activities of the cells, the time spent in minimally responsive A-level work style interactions, the amount of group resistance, and the percentage time of therapist participation in the group.

In our study (Kanas et al. 1985), a trained evaluator observed seven consecutive triweekly sessions of the schizophrenic group through a one-way mirror. During the 3-week evaluation period, 11 different male patients participated, and the average number of members per session was 5 patients and 2 therapists. Table 7–2 shows the results of the content and work style category scores in terms of their percentiles as applied to Hill's normative sample. As can be seen, our group fell in the typical range of the normative sample except for the confrontive category, which was at the 97th percentile. This is significant because it suggests that fewer than 3% of groups might be expected to exceed our group in this category. It is noteworthy that in the Hill system, the confrontive cate-

Table 7–2. HIM-G category scores (percentiles) for experimental groups versus Hill normative sample

Category	First inpatient study (Kanas et al. 1985)	Second inpatient study (Kanas and Smith 1990)	Outpatient group (Kanas and Smith 1990)
Content style			
Topic	75	68	70
Group	56	82	65
Relationship	49	58	60
Personal	43	26	34
Work style			
Confrontive	97	98	98
Assertive	64	68	60
Speculative	35	14	13
Conventional	34	48	52

Note. HIM-G is a form of the Hill Interaction Matrix.

gory represents the highest level of group work. According to the Hill Interaction Matrix Scoring Manual (Hill 1961), confrontive interactions are "characterized by a penetration to the significant aspects of a discussion; and because of this penetration, these statements confront members with aspects of their behavior usually avoided" (p. 54). Because true confrontation implies risk taking and honesty in interacting, not fault finding or attacking behavior (Hill 1965), an atmosphere of trust exists in groups high in this category. The most unique matrix cell was IE, which scored at the 99th+ percentile. The scoring manual (Hill 1961) states that "IE ratings are given to interaction in which discussions of pertinent topics about mental health or adjustment are synthesized or characterized in a penetrating and usually insightful fashion so that each member is personally confronted by the implications of the material being discussed" (p. 55).

Additional findings suggested that the group environment was safe and supported openness and trust. A-level interactions, which refer to no or minimal patient responses to a therapist's probing, occupied less than 1% of the group time, and group resistance occurred less than 1% of the time and never involved more than one group member per session. Specific category ratios indicated that participation was spread out among the members and that the members were open and assertive in stating their positions. The only instances of the Th/M ratio being above 1.00 was in the confrontive (E) category and in two of its cells (IIIE and IVE), which suggests that the therapists played an important role in shaping the most unique quality of this group: the tendency of the patients to be confronted about significant aspects of their illness. Overall, the therapists participated 10%–20% of the time.

To test the robustness of this treatment approach, we replicated the original HIM-G study 5 years later on the same unit but using a different rater, different patients, and different therapists (Kanas and Smith 1990). This time, 12 consecutive triweekly sessions consisting of 11 different male patients were evaluated, with an average session being composed of 5 patients and 2 therapists. Table 7–2 shows that the confrontive work style category again defined the uniqueness of the group, this time at the 98th percentile. Once again, matrix cell IE scored highest at the 99th+ percentile. The rank order of the 16 cells from this study was compared with the rank order from the original study using the

Spearman rank-order correlation. The results showed that the two rankings correlated significantly (rho = .66, $t = 3.29$, $P < .01$, two-tailed). Once again, the amount of minimally responsive A-level interactions and the total group resistance were low (each scoring at 1%–5% of overall group activity), and the therapists were moderately active (26% of the time). The highest Th/M category ratio (1.22) was found in the confrontive category, suggesting that the therapists were influential in shaping the uniqueness of this treatment approach. Thus, despite changes in staff and patient personnel, the environment of the group looked very much like that of the earlier group, supporting the robustness of the treatment model and suggesting that it can successfully be taught to new therapists.

In another inpatient study, we looked at the group process using the short form of the Group Climate Questionnaire (GCQ-S). This relatively new measure was developed by MacKenzie (1983, 1990) and consists of 12 statements that are rated on 7-point Likert scales after each session by either the patients or the therapists. Eleven of the scales are used to construct three group climate dimensions: engaged (an indicator of group cohesion), avoiding (an indicator of reluctance to face problems), and conflict (an indicator of interpersonal friction). The 12th scale is an indicator of general anxiety. The session dimension scores of a group can be averaged and compared with either patient or therapist means from a normative sample of 12 outpatient groups composed of neurotic and characterological patients. Although not as rigorous or widely used as the Hill Interaction Matrix, the GCQ-S has the advantages of being quick and easy to complete and of testing useful clinical constructs. In addition, changes in dimension scores from session to session can be plotted and compared with hypothetical changes that might indicate the presence of group stages (MacKenzie 1983, 1990; MacKenzie and Livesley 1983). As discussed in Chapter 6, however, this makes sense only in closed groups where the patient composition is relatively constant over time.

In this study (Kanas and Barr 1986), 34 consecutive sessions of our triweekly inpatient schizophrenic group were evaluated by the group leaders using the GCQ-S. Because a number of staff and trainees served as therapists during this time, we had to calculate interrater reliabilities, and these were at acceptable levels of significance for the three dimensions using the intraclass correlation coefficient. Because I attended all of the sessions as a cotherapist or as an observer behind a one-way mirror, I wrote down the topics that were discussed during the sessions, and these later were content analyzed. During the 3-month study period, 22 male patients participated in the group, and each session had an average number of 6 patients and 2 therapists. The GCQ-S mean dimension scores are shown in Table 7–3. There was no difference between our group and MacKenzie's (1983) normative sample in the avoiding dimension, but our group scored significantly lower in the engaged ($t = 2.53$, $P < .02$, two-tailed) and in the conflict ($t = 4.85$, $P < .001$, two-tailed) dimensions. The first finding was thought to be a reflection of the rapid patient turnover in this inpatient group and its disruptive influence on group cohesion, whereas the second finding was believed to be a reflection of the group techniques that encouraged safety and minimized the expression of interpersonal anger. MacKenzie does not report normative anxiety scale values, but our mean score of 2.58 would fall between the verbal descriptions of "somewhat" and "moderately" on the GCQ-S. Topics that related to encouraging contact with others were discussed most frequently during the 34 sessions, followed by issues related to the expression of emotions and to reality testing. Advice giving concerning medications or discharge plans was last in frequency.

Table 7–3. Group Climate Questionnaire (short form) mean dimension scores

Dimension	Veterans Administration inpatient study (Kanas and Barr 1986)	British inpatient study (N. Kanas, unpublished study, August 1994)	Short-term outpatient study (Kanas et al. 1989a)	Non-psychotic outpatient normative sample (MacKenzie 1983)
Engaged	12.79	16.80	14.86	14.61
Avoiding	9.74	5.70	7.66	10.33
Conflict	2.25	1.50	1.51	3.85

An unpublished process study (N. Kanas, August 1994) of an open inpatient schizophrenic group at a general hospital in a large city in England was conducted. I introduced the group model to the staff and participated as a co-therapist for half of the sessions. The patients were from two open units, each with 20 beds and each with an overall average length of stay of about 5 weeks. The group met twice weekly for 45-minute sessions. The first 10 sessions of the group's existence were evaluated using the GCQ-S. During this time, 12 male and 8 female patients participated. There were 10 blacks, 8 whites, and 2 patients of Asian descent. Each group session averaged 6 patients and 2 therapists. After each session, the two group leaders agreed on a consensus rating for the 12 GCQ-S statements and on the major topics that were discussed.

The three dimension scores are listed in Table 7–3. This group scored significantly higher than the VA inpatient group in the engaged dimension ($t = 2.65$, $P < .02$, two-tailed) and significantly lower in the avoiding dimension ($t = 3.53$, $P < .01$, two-tailed). Although the conflict score also was lower, this was not significant. The mean anxiety scale score of 1.30 also was significantly lower than the corresponding score (2.56) for the VA inpatient group ($t = 3.76$, $P < .001$, two-tailed). Thus, the British group seemed to be more cohesive and less avoidant and tense than the American group.

A number of factors may have contributed to these findings. First, the British group had a larger number of female patients (40%) than the VA group (0%). In general, female schizophrenic patients respond better to treatment than male schizophrenic patients (Szymanski et al. 1995). In most psychotherapy groups, it is believed that women are more supportive and emotionally expressive than men (Lazerson and Zilbach 1993), and there is some evidence that personal growth groups with women are more cohesive than all-male groups (Taylor and Strassberg 1986). Perhaps women play a similar role in schizophrenic groups using our model of treatment, thus accounting for the above results.

Second, sociocultural factors may have played a role. British patients may bond together differently than American VA patients. In addition, the fact that the members were diverse in their ethnic and social backgrounds may have led them to join together more around their common schizophrenic problems and symptoms. Also, the group was begun as the only psychotherapy group on the wards through the influence of a visiting professor from America. This may have enhanced its specialness, and the patients may have responded with unusual togetherness and openness.

Finally, although the average length of hospitalization was much longer in the British than in the American hospital, fewer group sessions were studied. This means that the patients comprising this group had less group experience during the evaluation period. For example, in the British group, 75% of the patients participated in one to three sessions, and none exceeded eight sessions. In contrast, in the VA group, 36% of the patients participated in one to three sessions, and half of them were involved in more than eight sessions. Thus, one could argue that in the British hospital, the GCQ-S was measuring a group that was less advanced, and this accounted for the different results. However, if this were true, one would expect the opposite findings: a less advanced group should be less cohesive and more avoidant than a group where the members had an opportunity to get to know one another for a longer period of time. Perhaps the patients had more time to interact out of the group on the longer-stay British wards, and this familiarity might have carried over into the group and increased its cohesion.

The relative influence of the factors described in explaining the GCQ-S findings cannot be resolved definitively by only two groups. Further studies are necessary to tease out the important issues.

The topics that were considered in the British group were reminiscent of those that were brought up in the VA group. Of the 26 topics that were recorded, 11 dealt with ways to cope with hallucinations and delusions, and 9 dealt with improving interpersonal relationships. Thus, the patients on both sides of the Atlantic discussed issues that were congruent with the group goals. The ward registrars and nurses learned the treatment model in a relatively brief period of time, and they and most of the patients indicated that the group was helpful.

Outpatient Studies

Encouraged by our early inpatient experiences, we applied the treatment model to the outpatient setting. Using the GCQ-S and a content analysis of discussion topics, we studied a schizophrenic group during the first 6 months of its existence at a psychiatric outpatient clinic that was associated with a university teaching hospital. The group met weekly for 1 hour, and 26 sessions were evaluated (Kanas et al. 1984). The group began with four members, but two additional members were added during session 5. After this, it was closed to new admissions. One patient left after session 23 when a promotion at work led to a scheduling conflict with the group. Throughout most of the study period, there were four male and two female patients; four were paranoid schizophrenic, and two had schizoaffective disorder. The two male therapists were third-year psychiatric residents. I was their supervisor and observed the sessions by sitting in the room but outside of the group circle. The patient attendance rate was 88%. The two group leaders independently completed the GCQ-S after each session, and they demonstrated a significant interrater reliability using the Pearson product-moment correlation.

The overall mean GCQ-S dimension scores did not differ significantly ($P < .05$) from the means in MacKenzie's (1983) outpatient normative sample, although the higher avoiding score just missed this level of significance. As was the case in our inpatient group (Kanas and Barr 1986), the anxiety score of 2.63 was between the verbal descriptions of "somewhat" and "moderately" on this scale.

Because the group was closed for most of its existence, we examined the session-by-session dimension scores to look for evidence of group developmental stages. There was a tendency for the engaged scores to increase and the conflict scores to decrease as time went on. During the final seven sessions, a pattern emerged where the engaged scores were high and the avoiding and conflict scores were low. In MacKenzie's system (MacKenzie 1983, 1990; MacKenzie and Livesley 1983), this pattern would be consistent with either a delayed stage 1, where the group finally is developing its identity and becoming cohesive, or with stage 3, where the members are attempting to achieve an understanding of their problems through self-revelation and introspection (see Chapter 6). However, these possibilities assume that outpatient groups of psychotic patients go through the same stage sequence as groups of neurotic and characterological patients. Our inability to find evidence of a typical developmental sequence earlier in the group suggests that this is not the case.

I recorded the topics that were discussed in this group. Issues related to the encouragement of contact with others were considered most frequently, followed by issues pertaining to reality testing, to the expression of emotions, and to advice giving, in that order.

Since the early 1980s, there has been much interest in short-term, time-limited therapy groups for nonpsychotic outpatients that typically meet for 8–16 sessions. Such groups are very cost-effective, and there is evidence that the mean number of sessions attended by most patients using group therapy is close to 8 (MacKenzie 1994). Furthermore, more than half of outpatients enrolled in different kinds of individual and group therapy improve in 8 or fewer sessions (MacKenzie 1990, 1994). Short-term therapy groups are characterized by careful patient selection, realistic goals, a clear focus, and directive therapists (Klein 1985). I became interested in using our approach in a format that treated schizophrenic patients in outpatient groups that met for 12 weekly 1-hour sessions. The goals were tightly regulated at helping the patients improve their relationships and learn ways of coping with their symptoms. The two therapists were supportive and actively encouraged the members to focus on these two goals in their discussions and to interact with each other during the sessions.

Our first study of this format was conducted at a university outpatient clinic (Kanas et al. 1988). I co-led the group with a third-year psychiatric resident. Seven patients began, but two dropped out by the third session. Of the five patients that completed the group, three were male; four were paranoid schizophrenic, and one had schizoaffective disorder. The attendance rate was 80%. The patients filled out several outcome measures before and after participating in the group, and at termination they completed the discharge questionnaire that we developed for an earlier study (Kanas and Barr 1982). A nurse-observer recorded the discussion topics. Four months after the group ended, the patients were contacted by phone and were asked several structured questions about their ability to relate with others, their ability to cope with psychotic experiences, and their treatment progress.

Although we found no significant pregroup–postgroup differences in symptoms as measured by the 90-item Symptom Checklist (SCL-90) or the Brief Psychiatric Rating Scale, there was a significant improvement in the predicted direction on the Social Avoidance and Distress Scale (SAD) ($t = 2.23, P < .05$, one-tailed). On the discharge questionnaire, all the members rated the group as being "very" or "somewhat" helpful. The rank order of therapeutic factors correlated significantly with the rank order from our earlier inpatient study (Kanas and Barr 1982) using the Spearman rank-order correlation (rho = .80, $t = 4.38, P < .01$, two-tailed). The members valued the group more for helping them learn to relate better with others and to test reality and cope with psychotic experiences than as a place to gain insight or to receive advice about their illness, medications, or economic situation (see Table 6–3 in Chapter 6). This paralleled the content analysis of discussion topics, which showed that relationship and reality-testing issues were discussed more often than issues related to advice giving, the group itself, or the expression of emotions.

During the structured telephone interviews 4 months after the group ended, four of the five patients reported gains in their ability to interact with other people, and two of them believed that they were coping better with psychotic experiences. None of the patients had been hospitalized or received any significant changes in their outpatient care. Two felt that their group experience was too short, and three said that it had been just right in length.

As a result of these encouraging findings, we decided to do a controlled study of our short-term, time-limited format at a VA outpatient clinic (Kanas et al. 1989b). Fourteen patients began one of two groups, and 12 of them finished. All of the completers were diagnosed as schizophrenic, and 11 of them were male. I co-led each group with a third-year psychiatric resident. The patient attendance rate for the two groups was 89%. Nine additional patients were assigned to a waiting list control condition, and they did not differ demographically from their counterparts in the groups. Both group and control patients were given the SCL-90 and the SAD initially and after completing their respective experimental condition (about 4 months for each). The discussion topics were recorded for both therapy groups. Finally, all patients were contacted 4 months later and asked a series of questions similar to those in the previous study.

On the SCL-90, the group patient scores dropped in all nine symptom dimensions. Two of these decreases (anxiety and somatization) were significant when compared with the waiting list patients using an analysis of variance. There was a nonsignificant decrease in group patient SAD scores. As in the previous study, topics dealing with relationships and coping with psychotic experiences were most frequently discussed, followed by issues pertaining to the therapy group itself, the expression of emotions, and advice giving.

In the 4-month follow-up interview, all of the group patients found their experience to be "very" or "somewhat" helpful. Three said it was too short, and nine thought it was about the right duration. Six indicated that they would like to be in a similar group in the future. When asked a series of questions about their clinical status, there were no significant interval changes using the Fisher exact test between the two conditions in terms of general psychological problems, antipsychotic medication dose, hospitalization status, outpatient therapy, living arrangements, job or disability status, legal status, or physical condition. As shown in Table 7–4, there were significant differences in two areas: relating with others and coping with psychosis (Kanas et al. 1989b). It is noteworthy that these are the two areas most congruent with the group goals and with the types of topics most often discussed in the sessions. This suggests that a short-term, time-limited therapy group for schizophrenic patients can have an impact for up to 4 months after the group ends in specific areas that are the focus of the discussions.

The university and the two VA groups described all were evaluated using the GCQ-S (Kanas et al. 1989a). The co-therapists

Table 7–4.   Significant 4-month interval questions

Question	Group patients (%)	Waiting list patients (%)	P
Relating better with other people	88	11	.01
Coping better with psychotic symptoms	63	0	.03

completed this measure after each session, and the interrater reliabilities for the three GCQ-S dimensions were at acceptable levels of significance using the intraclass correlation coefficient. The three groups did not differ from each other on any of the dimension scores, with the exception of one of the VA groups, which scored significantly higher than the other two in engaged. This unusually cohesive group also experienced no dropouts and had a much higher attendance rate (99%) than the other two. The patients in the three groups did not differ significantly in terms of sex, race, or diagnosis.

The composite mean dimension scores for the three groups are shown in Table 7–3. The groups did not differ from MacKenzie's (1983) outpatient normative sample in the engaged dimension, but they scored significantly lower in avoiding ($t = 7.03$, $P < .001$, two-tailed) and in conflict ($t = 6.88$, $P < .001$, two-tailed). The dimension scores varied high and low about the mean from session to session, and there was no evidence of sequential developmental stages (MacKenzie 1983; MacKenzie and Livesley 1983). Similar to the long-term group described earlier (Kanas et al. 1984), however, there was a tendency for the engaged scores to increase and the avoiding and conflict scores to decrease as time went on. The overall attendance rate of 86% (representing an average of five patients per session) and the low dropout rate of 19% suggested that the patients found the groups to be valuable enough to attend on a fairly regular basis.

Because many of the patients in the short-term groups indicated that they wanted another group experience, I decided to offer a "repeater's" group at the VA. The 12 VA-eligible patients who finished one of the earlier groups within the past 2 years were contacted, and 7 (58%) agreed to participate. One of these dropped out after the third session, and the remaining six (five men) completed it. Like its predecessors, the group consisted of 12 weekly 1-hour sessions and was closed to new admissions. Although the stated goals and topic areas were similar to the first groups, the repeater patients seemed to deal with relationship and symptom issues more efficiently than before and to discuss more sophisticated topics that included a recognition of long-standing maladaptive patterns of behavior. Each session averaged six patients and two therapists, and the patient attendance rate was 89%. At the end of the group, five members rated it as "very" helpful, and one said it was "somewhat" helpful.

Because the sessions of this group were videotaped, we had a trained rater score them using the HIM-G (Kanas and Smith 1990). Useful data were obtained on 11 of the sessions because there was no sound on the tape of session 8. Table 7–2 shows that the confrontive work style category again defined the uniqueness of the group at the 98th percentile. Also similar to the two previous inpatient studies (Kanas and Smith 1990; Kanas et al. 1985), matrix cell IE scored highest at the 99th+ percentile. Using the Spearman rank-order correlation, a ranking of the 16 matrix cells describing this group correlated significantly with both the first inpatient group (rho = .77, t = 4.52, P < .001, two-tailed) and the second inpatient group (rho = .90, t = 7.73, P < .001, two-tailed). Also similar to the findings from the two previous inpatient groups, the number of A-level interactions were relatively infrequent (scoring in the 5%–10% range), the total group resistance was low (1%–5% of overall group activity), and the therapists were moderately active overall (26% of the time). The highest Th/M category ratio (1.36) again was in the confrontive category, which once more suggested that the therapists were the primary contributors to the uniqueness of this group. Thus, in terms of the content and work constructs of the HIM-G, the environments of our short-term outpatient and inpatient groups are quite similar and support the notion that the treatment approach is effective and safe.

Summary of the Research Findings to Date

Based on those studies described that evaluated outcome, our integrative group therapy model is useful, safe, and oriented to the needs of schizophrenic patients. On questionnaires, both inpatients and outpatients rate their group experience as helpful. There is a suggestion that younger patients and nonparanoid schizophrenic patients benefit more from inpatient groups than their older and paranoid counterparts. Some outpatients experience symptom reduction and improvement in social anxiety, and they report improvement in relating with others and in coping with psychotic experiences up to 4 months after the group has ended. This is particularly notable because these two issues represent major therapeutic goals and generate the bulk of the discussion topics. More than half of the outpatients completing short-term groups may be expected to participate in a similar "repeater's" group within a year or two. Patients regularly come to the sessions: attendance rates typically are in the 80%–90% range. Finally, the outpatient dropout rates generally have been under 20%, and this compares favorably with one general review that reported group therapy dropout rates ranging from 25% to 57% (Yalom 1975).

Process studies suggest that in both inpatient and outpatient groups, the members are engaged in high-quality work that allows them to confront significant aspects of their problems. They respond to the therapists and to each other with minimal resistance, suggesting that they feel safe and are open in the sessions. On questionnaires, the patients indicate that they value the group more as a place to learn ways of interacting with others, to test reality and cope with schizophrenic symptoms, and to express feelings than as a place to gain insight and to receive guidance concerning their illness, medications, or economic situation. The therapists are active and successful in defining the unique parameters of the groups. In terms of content and work characteristics, new therapists can be taught the essence of the integrative model in both ward and clinic settings, suggesting that the approach is robust and replicable. The groups are relatively cohesive, and the members exhibit low levels of avoidance, conflict, and anxiety. Again, this suggests an environment that is interactive, open, and safe. Although there is little evidence of the kind of group stage development that occurs in outpatient groups of neurotic and characterological patients, the closed clinic groups demonstrate a pattern of increased cohesion and decreased avoidance and conflict as time goes on. Perhaps this is the kind of progression that one should expect in groups of psychotic patients.

The discussion topics are congruent with the group goals, which should not be surprising because these are made explicit and reinforced by the therapists. In both inpatient and outpatient groups, learning ways to interact better with others and to reality test and cope with schizophrenic symptoms are issues that are most frequently discussed. Advice giving around their illness, medications, or economic situation is least commonly considered by the patients. Topics related to emotions are intermediate in terms of frequency.

Although schizophrenia is a chronic mental illness that requires long-term follow-up and medication management, our results suggest that a short-term, time-limited group therapy approach can be useful. Where staffing and resources influence the use of this model, patients who need additional treatment can be accommodated in "repeater's" groups that are offered like psychological booster shots. Some patients will not find the group useful or will achieve maximal therapeutic benefit from just one course of treatment. For them, participating in a group that ends after 12 sessions will be enough and will give them the experience of dealing with loss and issues of termination. For others, being given the opportunity to be on their own and to try out new learning, while still knowing that they can join another group if the need arises, empowers them with control of their own destiny and prevents unnecessary treatment dependency. For still others who need more structure, regular attendance in sequential short-term groups or a long-term closed group might be the only practical solution. Thus, there is a place for both short-term and long-term groups for schizophrenic outpatients.

These conclusions are not the last word on the effectiveness and characteristics of the integrative group model. It would be desirable to examine and even to extend the model further in large-scale controlled studies at a number of different treatment settings and over longer periods of time (e.g., following patients for several years posttreatment). In addition, it would be useful to delineate further which schizophrenic patients benefit most from variations in the treatment approach (e.g., short-term versus long-term groups). Finally, the role of cultural factors and the influence of different male-to-female ratios on the group process would be important to study further. Although tight budgets and a bias toward biologically oriented studies have made it difficult to secure adequate funds to carry out such ambitious psychotherapy research projects during the past two decades, perhaps the funding climate will change in the future.

However, I believe that much has been learned from the studies that are presented here in terms of therapeutic outcome, group process, and discussion topics. The results support the value of the integrative approach, and they suggest that the specific needs of schizophrenic patients are being addressed. The group environment appears to be helpful, safe, and congruent with the treatment goals. In addition, one is comforted by the robustness and replicability of the findings across inpatient and outpatient settings and in different types of treatment delivery systems, both in the United States and abroad. Finally, the results from these studies have highlighted a number of important characteristics of the treatment model that make it easier to train students and clinicians who want to use this approach for their own patients.

References

Drake RE, Sederer LI: The adverse effects of intensive treatment of chronic schizophrenia. Compr Psychiatry 27:313–326, 1986

Geczy B, Sultenfuss J: Group psychotherapy on state hospital admission wards. Int J Group Psychother 45:1–15, 1995

Hill WF: Hill Interaction Matrix (HIM) Scoring Manual. Los Angeles, CA, Youth Studies Center, University of Southern California, 1961

Hill WF: Hill Interaction Matrix (HIM) Monograph. Los Angeles, CA, Youth Studies Center, University of Southern California, 1965

Kanas N, Barr MA: Short-term homogeneous group therapy for schizophrenic inpatients: a questionnaire evaluation. Group 6:32–38, 1982

Kanas N, Barr MA: Process and content in a short-term inpatient schizophrenic group. Small Group Behavior 17:355–363, 1986

Kanas N, Smith AJ: Schizophrenic group process: a comparison and replication using the HIM-G. Group 14:246–252, 1990

Kanas N, Rogers M, Kreth E, et al: Psychiatric research in a military setting: evolution of a study on inpatient group psychotherapy. Milit Med 143:552–555, 1978

Kanas N, Rogers M, Kreth E, et al: The effectiveness of group psychotherapy during the first three weeks of hospitalization: a controlled study. J Nerv Ment Dis 168:487–492, 1980

Kanas N, DiLella VJ, Jones J: Process and content in an outpatient schizophrenic group. Group 8:13–20, 1984

Kanas N, Barr MA, Dossick S: The homogeneous schizophrenic inpatient group: an evaluation using the Hill Interaction Matrix. Small Group Behavior 16:397–409, 1985

Kanas N, Stewart P, Haney K: Content and outcome in a short-term therapy group for schizophrenic outpatients. Hosp Community Psychiatry 39:437–439, 1988

Kanas N, Stewart P, Deri J, et al: Group process in short-term outpatient therapy groups for schizophrenics. Group 13:67–73, 1989a

Kanas N, Deri J, Ketter T, et al: Short-term outpatient therapy groups for schizophrenics. Int J Group Psychother 39:517–522, 1989b

Klein RH: Some principles of short-term group therapy. Int J Group Psychother 35:309–330, 1985

Lazerson JS, Zilbach JJ: Gender issues in group psychotherapy, in Comprehensive Group Psychotherapy, 3rd Edition. Edited by Kaplan HI, Sadock BJ. Baltimore, MD, Williams & Wilkins, 1993, pp 682–693

MacDonald WS, Blochberger CW, Maynard HM: Group therapy: a comparison of patient-led and staff-led groups on an open hospital ward. Psychiatr Q 38 (suppl):290–303, 1964

MacKenzie KR: The clinical application of a group climate measure, in Advances in Group Psychotherapy: Integrating Research and Practice. Edited by Dies RR, MacKenzie KR. New York, International Universities Press, 1983, pp 159–170

MacKenzie KR: Introduction to Time-Limited Group Psychotherapy. Washington, DC, American Psychiatric Press, 1990

MacKenzie KR: Where is here and when is now?: the adaptational challenge of mental health reform for group psychotherapy. Int J Group Psychother 44:407–428, 1994

MacKenzie KR, Livesley WJ: A developmental model for brief group therapy, in Advances in Group Psychotherapy: Integrating Research and Practice. Edited by Dies RR, MacKenzie KR. New York, International Universities Press, 1983, pp 101–116

Pattison EM, Brissenden E, Wohl T: Assessing special effects of inpatient group psychotherapy. Int J Group Psychother 17:283–297, 1967

Strassberg DS, Roback HB, Anchor KN, et al: Self-disclosure in group therapy with schizophrenics. Arch Gen Psychiatry 32:1259–1261, 1975

Szymanski S, Lieberman JA, Alvir JM, et al: Gender differences in onset of illness, treatment response, course, and biological indexes in first-episode schizophrenic patients. Am J Psychiatry 152:698–703, 1995

Taylor JR, Strassberg DS: The effects of sex composition on cohesiveness and interpersonal learning in short-term personal growth groups. Psychotherapy 23:267–273, 1986

Weiner MF: Outcome of psychoanalytically oriented group psychotherapy. Group 8:3–12, 1984

Yalom ID: The Theory and Practice of Group Psychotherapy, 2nd Edition. New York, Basic Books, 1975

CHAPTER 8

Conclusions

Schizophrenia is a serious mental illness that affects the content and process of thought. In terms of content, these patients experience hallucinations and delusions to the point of being psychotic. In terms of process, their thinking becomes disorganized in a variety of ways, such as being loose, circumstantial, or tangential. These disturbances in thought may be associated with problems involving affect, interpersonal relationships, sense of self, volition, and psychomotor behavior. Additional difficulties include problems with employment, education, finances, housing, self-care, and general quality of life.

Both biomedical and psychosocial treatment approaches are necessary. Although antipsychotic medications are a major treatment intervention, not all schizophrenic patients respond optimally to these drugs, and others do not take them on a regular basis due to serious side effects. Therefore, counseling; individual, group, and family therapy; and social services are important components of a complete biopsychosocial treatment plan. Given the characteristics of schizophrenia, group therapy would seem to be an especially valuable treatment modality, because its interpersonal nature presents a forum for these patients to share ways of coping with their symptoms, to gain support and test reality in the here and now of the sessions, and to improve their ability to relate with other people.

Historical and Theoretical Issues

Schizophrenic patients have been treated in therapy groups for more than 70 years. Clinical reports on this approach have been descriptive and optimistic in discussing the benefits of group therapy. Beginning with Lazell (1921), early reports focused on educative techniques and a lecture format, usually followed by a group discussion. Starting in the 1930s, psychoanalytic methods began to be used. Some authors cautioned that an insight-oriented, uncovering approach could be too stressful for psychotic patients, and they advocated including support and structure in the group. The 1950s saw the growth of interpersonal models that emphasized the relationship aspects of the disease and encouraged patients to interact in the here and now. During the past two decades, the educative, psychodynamic, and interpersonal approaches have continued to be used, but they often have been combined in more eclectic ways. In addition, specialized techniques have been introduced, such as those using Gestalt concepts, videotape playback, patient-led groups, and flexible drop-in formats.

To evaluate important trends more objectively, I conducted a literature review of controlled studies that involved therapy groups with schizophrenic patients. The review dated back to the time that antipsychotic medications began to be used in the clinical setting, and it spanned more than 40 years from 1950 to 1991. All studies compared at least one group therapy condition with a no-group therapy control condition, had at least 50% schizophrenic patients or partialed out the effects of the groups on schizophrenic patients, included at least one major outcome measure, and stated the duration of treatment. The 46 studies were rated in terms of whether they concluded that group therapy was significantly more effective, no different from, or less effective than the control condition. The studies were categorized in terms of being inpatient or outpatient and in terms of being long, intermediate, or short in duration. In addition, the 57 groups involved in the studies were classified as being insight oriented, interaction oriented, or other/unspecified in an attempt to see if any one of these clinical approaches was more beneficial than the others.

The results of the review found that group therapy was effective for schizophrenic patients in both inpatient and outpatient settings. Overall, 70% of the studies found that it was significantly better than the no-group therapy control condition, and it was as effective or more effective than individual therapy for schizophrenic patients in those studies that made this comparison. There was a tendency for long-term inpatient groups (i.e., lasting longer than 36 sessions) to be more effective than short- or intermediate-term groups. Insight-oriented approaches that emphasized uncovering and psychodynamic issues were significantly less effective than interaction-oriented approaches that emphasized interpersonal problems and relationship issues in the here and now. This especially was true in the inpatient setting. In fact, insight-oriented techniques were harmful for some schizophrenic patients in inpatient groups. These patients seemed to be better off having unstructured time on the ward than participating in a treatment modality that was probably too intense for their fragile egos.

Theoretically, there have been three traditional approaches: the educative, the psychodynamic, and the interpersonal. The educative approach emphasizes the biological and phenomenological aspects of schizophrenia. Consequently, the groups using this model of treatment try to help the members learn to cope with the symptoms of the illness and to deal with the real problems that these symptoms cause. Typical techniques include lectures, advice giving, question-and-answer periods, problem solving, role-playing, and homework assignments between the sessions. The time focus is on the current manifestations and sequelae of the disease. This approach imparts cognitive information that gives the patients a sense of control and mastery over their symptoms, and the didactic format provides a structured, safe group environment. Biomedical coping strategies are emphasized, such as taking additional medication to relieve stress. Although the discussions that follow the presentations allow the members to interact and share ideas, the content usually relates to a specific agenda item for that session, and this makes it difficult for the group to consider other issues that may be more immediate for some of the members.

The psychodynamic approach emphasizes the psychological aspects of schizophrenia. The goals are to help the members understand how long-term psychological problems and maladaptive behaviors interfere with their lives, with the hope of lessening the impact of these difficulties and improving ego functions. Techniques include discussions where topics are generated by the patients, the uncovering of important unconscious issues, and interpretations of transference. The time focus is on the past antecedents of the disease and the ways in which they have affected a patient's current situation. This model can be very intensive because unpleasant material may be discovered, and this may result in anxiety, regression, and exacerbation of symptoms. In addition, like the educative model, relatively little attention is paid to member interactions during the sessions and the ways in which they can be used to help the patients relate better with each other and with people outside of the group.

This last problem is corrected in the interpersonal approach, which places great importance on the relationship aspects of schizophrenia. The goals of these groups are to help the members become less socially isolated and to improve their ability to interact with other people. Techniques include facilitating open discussions of interpersonal problems, encouraging patients to relate with each other during the sessions using a variety of techniques (e.g., structured exercises, reinforcing patient-to-patient eye contact), and interpreting maladaptive interactions that are observed in the group. The time focus is the present, and this includes both the here and now of the sessions as well as each patient's current life outside of the group. However, like too much uncovering, intensive work in the here and now can make patients anxious, particularly if interpersonal anger is involved. Also, the use of structured exercises to encourage interactions is not necessary for most schizophrenic patients, and these exercises may infantilize the patients and take time away from other issues that need to be discussed.

As a result of a series of clinical research projects by me and my colleagues, a treatment model for treating schizophrenic patients in therapy groups, which I call the integrative approach, has been developed. In its evolution over time, it has taken on a biopsychosocial perspective that allows it to be compared with the three treatment models described. Like the educative approach, it helps patients learn ways of coping with psychotic symptoms (although psychosocial strategies are given more emphasis than medication strategies). Also, discussion topics are related to the specific needs of these patients. Finally, although patient safety is similarly enhanced by the structure of the group, this structure is not built into the format but instead is provided through the interventions of the therapists.

Like the psychodynamic approach, the integrative groups use open discussions where the members generate the topics. Similarly, lectures and formal structured exercises are not a major part of this model, although the go-around technique is employed at times, and there is a brief orientation whenever a new member is added. Long-term problems also may be examined, especially in the outpatient setting, but the major focus is how these past conflicts and maladaptive behaviors currently affect the patients. Finally, ego functions are strengthened in the groups, particularly reality testing and reality sense.

Like the interpersonal approach, a major goal of the integrative model is to help the members become less isolative and improve their relationships. This is done through the discussions as well as through the experiences the patients have in interacting with each other during the sessions. Techniques are used to encourage these member interactions, and when they are maladaptive, the therapist will diplomatically intervene in the here and now, with the intent of giving the patients immediate feedback on ways in which they can relate more appropriately.

Clinical Issues

There are two major goals in the integrative group approach. The first aims to help the members learn how to cope with their symptoms. For the majority of patients, this means learning to test reality and deal with psychotic symptoms, such as hallucinations and delusions. The second goal of treatment is to help the patients learn how to improve their interpersonal relationships. This is done through the discussions as well as through the experience of interacting with others in the group.

In open groups on acute-care inpatient units, the main focus is to help the members deal with their psychotic symptoms, and interpersonal problems usually are considered in reference to the psychotic state. In closed outpatient groups that are newly formed or are short term, discussions usually focus on both symptoms and interpersonal issues. After a closed group has met for some time and the patients have learned to cope with their symptoms, issues concerning relationships tend to dominate, and longstanding problems and maladaptive behaviors are discussed with reference to their impact on current functioning. The overwhelming majority of patients in the groups have a diagnosis of schizophrenia, although a few suffer from related conditions: schizophreniform, schizoaffective disorder, and delusional disorder. This high degree of homogeneity allows the groups to be cohesive and the therapists to utilize techniques that are useful for these patients while also avoiding those that are too intensive and produce anxiety and regression. Patients who suffer from severe positive symptoms or from negative symptoms also can be treated as long as they are directable and can tolerate staying in the group for the whole session. Heterogeneous groups consisting of both schizophrenic and nonschizophrenic patients may be conducted in the outpatient setting if the patients are stable and if the format is supportive and focuses on current problems. High-functioning patients and those with memory deficits gain little from the integrative groups. Also, acutely manic or antisocial patients only disrupt the process and create an antitherapeutic environment for all of the members.

The groups have been conducted in both inpatient and outpatient settings at a variety of locations, and they have ranged from short-term (e.g., 12 sessions) to long-term in duration. Adults of both genders and all races, ages, and backgrounds have been treated. Especially in stable outpatient settings where the members discuss long-term problems and maladaptive relationships, it is useful to include both men and women and people of different cultural backgrounds in the group.

A co-therapy approach has several advantages. Groups of psychotic patients can be chaotic at times, and it is easier for two therapists to maintain control and deal with unsafe situations than it is for one therapist. Two leaders also can model nonpsychotic interactions and provide more feedback in reality-testing situations. When a therapist is on vacation or is ill, the group still can be held if the patients are stable enough for the remaining leader to handle. Finally, a co-therapy approach can help alleviate the stress and potential for burnout that can result from leading groups with psychotic patients. Although it is ideal for the same two therapists to lead all of the sessions, in the inpatient setting staff turnover and schedule changes make this difficult. In this situation, it is necessary to have a pool of trained leaders who substitute for each other depending on staff availability. Male-female co-therapy teams are useful but not critical in groups of psychotic patients. The professional backgrounds of the therapists are not important, as long as both are well trained to do the group and are seen as being equally active and helpful by the patients.

The inpatient groups are open and usually meet for 45 minutes three times a week, although daily groups are useful if staff availability allows. Sessions are not held with fewer than 3 patients, and more than 8 make the group hard to manage. The ideal patient range is 5–7. In the outpatient setting, the groups are closed and meet for 60 minutes once a week, although this frequency can be increased in some settings (e.g., day treatment programs). To account for dropouts, the groups usually start with 8–10 patients, and an average attendance of 6–8 is optimal.

Most of the patients receive antipsychotic medications, and this is quite compatible with the groups. The use of group time to discuss medication dosage and side effects is discouraged, although feelings about having to take medications and the value of these drugs in coping with psychotic experiences are appropriate discussion topics. Where possible, patient-to-patient feedback on medications is encouraged rather than advice giving from the therapists. Members who have technical questions or concerns about their prescriptions are referred back to their physicians.

The therapists should be active and directive in keeping the members focused on the topic. Their interventions need to be clear, consistent, and concrete, and it never hurts to repeat important statements in groups consisting of psychotic patients. Comments need to be made supportively and diplomatically, and the therapists should be open and willing to give their opinions about important matters. Discussions that focus on the here and now are more productive than those that focus on the there and then.

Discussion topics should meet the needs of the patients. Examples of helpful topics are auditory hallucinations; persecutory, referential, and grandiose delusions; thought insertion and thought broadcasting; disorganized thinking; relations with others; and emotional themes that typically are well tolerated by the group members, such as loneliness, depression, and despair.

Therapist-to-patient advice is not an ideal use of group time and should be used primarily to give support, structure the sessions, and advance the discussion topics. Patient-to-patient feedback is more productive, because it stimulates group interactions and encourages the members to share coping strategies with each other.

Any topic that produces anxiety can cause regression and an intensification of symptoms in schizophrenic patients. Caution needs to be exercised around issues related to anger, aggression, and sexual orientation or identity. Issues that reveal unconscious conflicts and flood the members with painful insights are also to be avoided in groups of psychotic patients.

Topics may be developed by discussing them in general terms first and then applying them personally to the group members or by asking all of the patients to comment on an issue through a go-around. A typical session proceeds by identifying an appropriate topic for discussion, then generalizing it to all the members, and finally asking them to share coping strategies. These strategies often cluster into one of two major areas: decreasing the amount of stress in the patients' lives or providing more stimulation when their environment is impoverished.

During the first session of a closed group, the goals and ground rules are explained, and the patients discuss their problems and what they hope to accomplish during the sessions. During the last session, the patients state their feelings about termination and indicate what they got out of the group before saying their goodbyes. The go-around technique can be used to make sure that all of the members participate in these two special sessions.

Patients who are being evaluated for admission to an ongoing open group need to be oriented to the goals and ground rules before they begin. At the start of their first session, they are told the kinds of issues that are discussed by the continuing members, and they are asked to share which of these issues are problematic for them. In this way, new members see that they are not alone with their problems, and they are quickly integrated into the group. Time also is provided to say goodbye to members who are being discharged. Patients who terminate through death or illness can distress the remaining members, and the therapists need to provide an opportunity for the latter to discuss their feelings and concerns openly.

Some schizophrenic patients benefit from concurrent group and individual therapy. Individual approaches have varied from traditional one-to-one, discussion-oriented supportive therapy to specialized approaches that teach social skills or help the patients learn ways of coping with psychotic experiences using behavioral and educational techniques. In several reviews, group and individual therapy are about equally effective, although the former is more cost-effective. With a given patient, however, there are pros and cons to each approach, and sometimes both treatments are indicated to deal with all of the problems that are presented.

The therapists need to be sensitive to the group dynamics. When an individual member is having a problem, he or she may become the focus of the discussion. When two members relate maladaptively, their interaction can become the topic for a session. When three or more people are affected in a similar manner by something that is being said or done, the therapists should consider that everyone is involved to some degree, and they can intervene at the group level. Thus, the interactions of the members in the here and now are not only powerful change factors, but they also give clues into the group dynamics and can influence the therapists' interventions.

When the members are interacting productively around topics that are related to the needs of schizophrenic patients, the therapists should remain quiet. However, when the group members are disorganized and cannot remain on a topic, or when the members are quiet or discussing irrelevant issues, the therapists can intervene to provide structure or to help the patients focus on an issue. When the environment is tense or unsafe, the therapists should change the subject or comment on the potential for danger and suggest a break in the discussion.

The integrative model has been used in a variety of inpatient and outpatient settings in the United States and abroad. Although social, cultural, and language issues affect the group process, the groups generally can keep on track and accomplish their clinical goals. Highly cohesive groups have resulted, as the members find a way to bond together around their common illness despite political adversity and demographic diversity.

The treatment model has been taught to a number of mental health staff and trainees. The ideal training module for ongoing inpatient groups includes didactic presentations and readings, observations of previous sessions on videotape, and direct viewings of current sessions through a one-way mirror or seated in the room outside of the group circle. The one-way mirror scenario allows the trainees to discuss the group in real time with a supervisor, and it offers a nonintrusive observational format that is well received by the patients as long as they have been introduced to the people who will be watching. Observing trainees, supervisors, and therapists participate in a rehash after each session. When a trainee is ready to begin, he or she is paired with a more experienced staff member as a co-therapist. In closed outpatient groups, a trainee may lead the group with a more experienced co-therapist for long periods of time. It is important for both leaders to participate and to be seen as equally helpful by the members. Common supervisory issues relate to the amount of activity the trainee displays and the need for interventions to be short, concrete, and clear.

Like many other therapy groups, our integrative groups are useful and cost-effective. Patients receive help for their symptoms and for their interpersonal problems, and there is a high rate of attendance in these groups. Inpatients value their experience and are amenable to participating in similar groups as outpatients, which improves their clinical course. The staff-to-patient ratio is on the order of 1:3 or 1:4. For many patients, participation in the groups obviates the need for more staff-intensive individual therapy, because they learn to relate better with others during the sessions and because group therapy for schizophrenic patients has been found to be as effective as or more effective than individual therapy in controlled studies. Finally, short-term groups that are based on the integrative model have been found to be safe and beneficial. In the outpatient setting, these represent a less expensive alternative to long-term group therapy, because nearly half of the patients believe that one 12-week trial is enough, and they do not feel the need to request a second group experience.

Research Issues

The integrative group therapy model described in this book has been empirically developed and supported by a number of outcome, process, and content studies dating back to 1975. These studies have taken place in a variety of inpatient and outpatient settings. In terms of outcome, the approach has been found to be useful, safe, and oriented to the needs of schizophrenic patients. The members have rated their group experience as being helpful at the time of discharge, with younger and nonparanoid patients being more positive than older and paranoid patients. Some outpatients have reported symptom reduction and improvement in social anxiety, as well as improvement in relating with others and in coping with psychotic experiences for up to 4 months after the group has ended. More than half of the outpatients who have completed a short-term, 12-session group choose to participate in a similar group within a year or two. Attendance rates are in the 80%–90% range, and dropout rates are less than 20%.

Studies of the group process suggest that, in both inpatient and outpatient settings, the members are engaged in high-quality work that allows them to confront significant aspects of their problems with minimal resistance and anxiety. The patients value the groups more as a place to learn ways of interacting better with others, to test reality and cope with schizophrenic symptoms, and to express feelings than as a place to gain insight and to receive advice concerning their illness, medications, or economic situation. The therapists are active and successful in defining the unique parameters of the groups. New therapists can reliably be taught the group model, suggesting that the approach is robust and replicable. The groups are cohesive, and the members exhibit low levels of avoidance, conflict, and anxiety. Although there is little evidence of the kind of stage development that occurs in closed groups of neurotic and characterological patients, the outpatient integrative groups show a pattern of increased cohesion and decreased avoidance and conflict as time goes on.

The topics that are discussed are congruent with the group goals. In both inpatient and outpatient settings, learning ways of interacting better with others and testing reality and coping with schizophrenic symptoms are most frequently discussed. Advice giving around their illness, medications, or economic situation are least commonly considered by the group members. Topics related to emotions are intermediate in terms of frequency.

Time-limited groups lasting for 12 sessions have been found to be useful and practical for schizophrenic outpatients. For those who find that one course of treatment is enough, the opportunity to terminate a therapeutic activity successfully boosts their confidence, gives them the experience of dealing with loss, and prevents unnecessary treatment dependency. For those who need more structure, regularly being able to attend sequential short-term "repeater's" groups or a long-term closed group presents the patients with viable treatment options.

Future research directions involving the integrative model include examining its effectiveness in controlled studies using long-term follow-up, delineating which patients benefit most from variations in the treatment model (e.g., short- versus long-term groups), and exploring further the role of cultural factors and different male-to-female ratios on the group process. But the results of more than 20 years of clinical and empirical work to date support the notion that the integrative group therapy approach presented in this book is helpful, safe, and relevant to the needs of schizophrenic patients when used in conjunction with antipsychotic medications. The model can be taught to others in a relatively brief period of time. It also has shown great applicability across inpatient and outpatient settings and in different types of treatment delivery systems, both in the United States and abroad. Thus, this approach is an important addition to the armamentarium of treatments that are available to meet the needs of schizophrenic patients.

Reference

Lazell EW: The group treatment of dementia praecox. Psychoanal Rev 8:168–179, 1921

Index

Page numbers printed in **boldface** *type refer to tables.*